Tobacco Use and Intimate Relationships

Ian Newman · John DeFrain

Tobacco Use and Intimate Relationships

Smokers and Non-Smokers Tell Their Stories

palgrave
macmillan

Ian Newman
University of Nebraska–Lincoln
Lincoln, NE, USA

John DeFrain
University of Nebraska–Lincoln
Lincoln, NE, USA

ISBN 978-3-030-06465-5 ISBN 978-3-319-92579-0 (eBook)
https://doi.org/10.1007/978-3-319-92579-0

Softcover re-print of the Hardcover 1st edition 2018

Printed on acid-free paper

This Palgrave Macmillan imprint is published by the registered company Springer International Publishing AG part of Springer Nature
The registered company address is: Gewerbestrasse 11, 6330 Cham, Switzerland

Preface

How does tobacco use really affect the lives of individuals and families? That simple question led us on a long journey of understanding. With the help of smokers and nonsmokers in every corner of America who spent many hours telling their stories in great detail, we believe we now have a much better picture of the challenges faced.

What they told us is well worth sharing: the precise dynamic of how smoking affects couple relationships and parent–child relationships; how anger, silence, and secrecy are wrapped up in the smoking dynamic; the battle in the home behind closed doors as both smokers and nonsmokers invoke personal rights and the American way in efforts to win arguments and defend positions; the intimate, behind-the-scenes private and personal discussions over health and the effects of smoking on smokers and nonsmokers; how smoking controls one's life in many ways, controlling when and where a smoker can find a place to smoke without retaliation and where nonsmokers can find a smoke-free environment.

And, by far the most important of all, we learned how absolutely essential communication is—how smokers and their loved ones will never be at peace until they find a way to speak courageously and honestly from the heart, and, even more important, until they find a way to listen to each other from the heart and genuinely understand what each is saying. Reading the many stories in this book from lifelong smokers, unrepentant smokers, smokers who can't quit, smokers who don't want to quit, former smokers, and lifelong nonsmokers gives us a broad and deep understanding of how the controversy that has raged in the media is really fought behind closed doors.

Reading this positive, objective, nonjudgmental book is a step in the right direction, a way out of the dilemma. Positive communication among couples and families leads to a better understanding of each other. This, in turn, leads to respect and appreciation for each other's needs, which leads to more fulfilling lives together.

Lincoln, USA

Ian Newman
John DeFrain

Acknowledgements

Jocelyn Herstein at the University of Nebraska Medical Center College of Public Health searched the literature for background material on many aspects of tobacco use. Ardis Holland, Cindy Jeffrey, Judy Martin, Phyllis Fogerty, and Betty Olson read early versions of this manuscript and provided helpful suggestions. Aimee Allard, graduate student in the Department of English at University of Nebraska–Lincoln, proofread the manuscript. Any spelling and grammar errors that may have crept into the subsequent revisions are not her fault. Michelle Maas, research project assistant at the Nebraska Center for Alcohol and Drug Abuse, University of Nebraska–Lincoln College of Education and Human Sciences, served as the research and clerical assistant throughout the project and provided insightful suggestions to keep the text focused on its original purpose. Over many years, Tagi Qolouvaki, a member of the English faculty at Hawai'i Community College in Hilo, Hawai'i, has shared her experiences as a smoker, former smoker and growing up in a home with smokers, providing invaluable insights throughout this project. Her experiences and skills as an insightful reader and analyst in reading testimony helped guide the development of the themes of this book.

Most importantly, to the hundreds of people who responded to our invitation and to the 139 who completed a questionnaire and mailed it back to us—whether you wrote dozens of words or dozens of pages—thank you for your trust, candor, and courage.

Quotes

"A smoker is not being fair to their family."—A Former Smoker

"He wouldn't accept the fact that smoking was turning me off." —A Former Smoker

"I smoke. It makes no sense!"—A Smoker Who Can't Quit

"I feel hateful toward my mother."—A Former Smoker

"I do not want to be part of her slow, painful death."—A Former Smoker

"I have a serious addiction."—An Unrepentant Smoker

"It's so unhealthy and I want him to live."—A Lifelong Nonsmoker

"Actually, I loved every aspect of smoking."—A Former Smoker

"I've always enjoyed smoking and could stop if I wished to."—An Unrepentant Smoker

"Smoking is more enjoyable than eating."—An Unrepentant Smoker

"I have never seen a tobacco ad show a person with emphysema." —A Smoker Who Won't Quit

"I hate everything about smoking, but I love to smoke and I can't stop!"—A Smoker Who Can't Quit

"I chased this guy, threatening to brain him with my crutches." —A Former Smoker

"I was smoking up to three packs a day, depending on my level of boredom:"—A Former Smoker

"Smokers have a hard road to travel." —A Former Smoker

"There is not one cigarette that I do not enjoy or look forward to." —A Smoker Who Can't Quit

"It's almost like ecstasy when I light up." —An Unrepentant Smoker

"More than likely I will not see my grandchildren grow up."—A Former Smoker

"My doctor told my husband I was a human time bomb."—A Former Smoker

"It is difficult to do this, to bring back all the bad memories, but here goes…"—A Former Smoker

"I would do anything to get one."—A Former Smoker

"My whole adult life has revolved around smoking."—A Smoker Who Can't Quit

"Not only was he a victim of tobacco—so were we."—A Former Smoker

"I consider quitting to be one of the greatest accomplishments of my life."—A Former Smoker

Contents

CHAPTER 1

Introduction

How does tobacco use really affect the lives of individuals and families? That simple question led us on a long journey of understanding. With the help of 225 smokers and nonsmokers in every corner of America who spent many hours telling their stories in great detail, we believe we now have a much better picture of the challenges faced.

What they told us is well worth sharing: the precise dynamic of how smoking affects couple relationships and parent–child relationships; how anger, silence, and secrecy are wrapped up in the smoking dynamic; the battle in the home behind closed doors as both smokers and nonsmokers invoke personal rights and the American way in efforts to win arguments and defend positions; the intimate, behind-the-scenes private and personal discussions over health and the effects of smoking on smokers and nonsmokers; how smoking controls one's life in many ways, controlling when and where a smoker can find a place to smoke without retaliation and where nonsmokers can find a smoke-free environment.

And, by far the most important of all, we learned how absolutely essential positive communication is—how smokers and their loved ones will never be at peace until they find a way to speak courageously and honestly from the heart, and, even more important, until they find a way to listen to each other from the heart and genuinely understand what each is saying. Positive communication aims at building bonds between individuals and making it possible to work together toward common goals. Rather than lining up against each other and struggling toward some kind of false victory, one side over the other, smokers and

I. Newman and J. DeFrain, *Tobacco Use and Intimate Relationships*,
https://doi.org/10.1007/978-3-319-92579-0_1

nonsmokers can unite in their families and find ways so that they can live more happily together.

Reading the many stories in this book from lifelong smokers, unrepentant smokers, smokers who can't quit, smokers who don't want to quit, former smokers, and lifelong nonsmokers gives us a broad and deep understanding of the controversy that has raged in the media and that is really fought behind closed doors.

The reader quickly sees how many people really are not listening to each other and can, thus, doom themselves to playing out their lives like an endless and hopeless TV political discussion. All this may seem entertaining on TV, but in reality, it is terribly demoralizing.

Reading this positive, objective, nonjudgmental book is a step in the right direction, a way out of the dilemma. Communication leads to a better understanding of each other, which leads to respect and appreciation for each other's needs, which leads to more fulfilling lives together.

Each of the stories you will read in this book is, as nearly as possible, the original words of the people who chose to talk candidly about the social, physical, and psychological impact of tobacco use on themselves and their families. The authors have changed names, dates, locations, and other details that might identify individual respondents, in order to protect their privacy. For information on the methods used in this project, please turn to the Appendices.

CHAPTER 2

Marital and Couple Relationships

Tobacco use significantly affects and can determine the shape of all familial relationships. Given the complexity of family relationships and range of family types, we will limit our examination here to how tobacco use affects two types of familial relationships in particular: marital and couple relationships and parent–child relationships. Tobacco use influences each of these types of relationships in significantly different ways. However, many of the key issues in both types of relationships are the same: the need for trust, intimacy, respect, and communication.

Since the family often includes couple and parent–child relationships, the effects of tobacco use on each of the relationships are complicated by the complex interconnections of the family unit as a whole. Furthermore, in regard to experiences as a child in one's family or origin can influence the relationships of adult partners with tobacco and consequently shape their own familial relationships with their children. After all, the path of least resistance is to practice as adults what we learn as children.

Smoking invariably influences couple relationships in many ways. For the nonsmoking partner (or the partner who has quit), issues of trust and intimacy are paramount. Many nonsmoking correspondents describe feeling betrayed when partners smoke in secret, or pretend to have quit smoking. Nonsmoking partners are also apt to suffer stress over the physical, emotional, and financial effects of smoking on their family as a whole. Finally, nonsmoking partners who experience the illness or death of a partner due to smoking must undergo the emotional, physical,

I. Newman and J. DeFrain, *Tobacco Use and Intimate Relationships*,
https://doi.org/10.1007/978-3-319-92579-0_2

and psychological stress of caregiving in addition to the loss of a partner. The knowledge that illness, disfigurement, or death could have been prevented can lengthen and aggravate the grief process for survivors of loved ones.

On the other hand, the smoking spouse/partner must deal with feelings of guilt and shame if they believe that their habit or addiction is harmful to their partners and other family members. Unfortunately, as revealed by much of their testimony, the pressure from loved ones to quit only increases the intensity of feelings smokers already have, inflating their sense of failure and humiliation. This can lead initially to increased use of tobacco. Smokers who admit the dangers of tobacco use also report stress about prematurely leaving their partners and families without adequate means of support due to smoking-related illness, in addition to fear for the health of their loved ones and themselves.

Further, because smoking often becomes an issue of rights and choice, to smoke or not smoke may be a threat to individual autonomy and equality within the relationship. For example, female partners who smoke may feel that their right to smoke should not be a right their male spouse can revoke, and male partners may feel publicly humiliated when their spouse and children "scold" them about their habit and pressure them to quit. These emotions only exacerbate the problems of smoking in families and do not lend themselves to what is so essential for both smoking and nonsmoking family members—communication, empathy, and support.

Tobacco use also affects marital/partner intimacy. Many nonsmokers, including those who have quit, speak to the difficulties of intimacy with a smoking spouse because of the physical effects of tobacco use—the smell of tobacco on the breath, hair, skin, and clothing of their partners. Additionally, some partners point to smoking and smoking-related illness as the cause of diminished libido and impotence for their smoking spouse/partner. Nonsmoking partners may be so repulsed by the physical effects of tobacco use on their spouse/partner that they lose the desire for intimacy and become physically and emotionally estranged; some contemplate divorce. For the nonsmoker, a partner's secret smoking or broken promises to quit may foster feelings of betrayal that lead to a loss of trust. Some nonsmoking spouses do not understand how their partners cannot quit a habit that endangers their own health and threatens their relationships. As with other marital/relationship problems, lack of desire for intimacy, loss of trust and communication, and anger about the dangers of secondhand smoke, all of which a nonsmoker may experience with a smoking spouse/partner, can lead to further estrangement, the internalization of guilt for dissolution of the relationship: "it was my fault," and divorce.

It is difficult for both smokers and nonsmokers to understand each other's needs and fears. The nonsmoker believes that if their partner really cared, they would make the effort to quit. The smoker feels constantly misunderstood and under pressure to quit; besides, it is not easy to kick an addiction. But while the issues surrounding smoking in a marriage are heavily emotional, communication often deteriorates into unproductive arguments; a nonsmoker's fear for his spouse's well-being turns into disgust and "nagging" and a smoker's inability to quit become insidious secret smoking.

Testimony

My present husband has allergies and smoking bothers him. Smoking bothers my mother-in-law. I just say you have to take me the way I am, even though deep inside I would like to quit smoking. It doesn't make me feel good. I am tired all the time. (a smoker who can't quit)

*****

My sister's house was in a constant state of tension for two years as she struggled to quit. Her husband and seven-year-old daughter put tremendous pressure on her. She smoked when they were not around. She resented the pressure and hated herself for sneaking. (a former smoker)

*****

I met my second husband about five years ago and did not realize, even after we married, that he had been a smoker for years and only quit cold turkey eight years earlier! He had smoked since he was about eighteen. We were married six months when I saw him on the porch hiding a cigarette from me. I never even considered that he might smoke. He stopped hiding it shortly after I saw him that first time, and expressed sorrow and guilt that he had started again. I noticed that his teeth yellowed faster and that he had a lingering odor that even a shower and mouthwash couldn't get rid of. I mentioned kindly that the smell offended me and turned me off at night. I was careful not to insult him for his habit; I wanted to prevent upset in the family for this minor irritation. I wouldn't divorce him for it; but it sure could be a source of friction that could gnaw at you until you let it out over something that might not even be related. (a former smoker)

*****

My husband and I feel fortunate that we were able to celebrate our recent anniversary. Had I not insisted that Frank see a doctor, a few months would have made all the difference. There is no doubt in our minds that had he waited he would not be here now, or if he had lived, the quality of his life would have been changed dramatically. There is no doubt whatsoever that years of cigarette smoking were the cause of his cancer. Our children have suffered with us. (a former smoker)

*****

Just prior to the cancer diagnosis, my marriage had been very strained. I had established a small business for my wife as a hedge against the very possibility that I might be incapacitated; I wanted her to have "a way to go" if I was unable to continue to support her, or if we separated. The hospital was 185 miles away, I was thought to be dying, and she had her business to maintain, which was her sole livelihood. She could only visit an average of twice a week. The feeling of abandonment was devastating! (a former smoker)

*****

I encouraged my spouse to try whatever was available to quit smoking. However, I did not like being with him when he was trying to quit. It's not an easy time. He cheats—hiding behind trees even. Now I say, "Keep smoking, but don't take it out on me. End your life sooner, that's your choice." We've gone through the process many times and he always goes back to smoking. (a nonsmoker)

*****

My husband of almost 51 years is still on his feet at 94. He has breathed secondhand smoke half a century with me without so much as an allergy. He did develop bladder stones and gallbladder stones after he was 90, but no prostate cancer. ***Will I kill him someday with my smoke?*** *(a smoker who can't quit)*

*****

...I married for the third time, to a woman who smokes. Well, now I can't breathe in my own home. I refuse to hug her for the stench of cigarettes in her hair, her breath stinks, and we now sleep in separate rooms after only five years of marriage. (a former smoker)

*****

Husband number two nagged me quite a bit about smoking, but I needed my friendly cigarettes to get by. I never really had what you would call a stable home life. ***In smoking I found something that I could count on and control, and no one was going to take that away.*** *(a smoker who can't quit)*

*****

My wife and three children have been strongly opposed to my smoking for several years, and I have not smoked in the presence of my children for at least the past five years. I continue to smoke in the presence of my wife, over her objections and constant reminders that it is extremely detrimental to my health. Obviously I recognize that I have a serious addiction. (an unrepentant smoker)

*****

Stories

A Smoker Is Not Being Fair to Their Family—A Former Smoker

My wife passed away in May of this year, and I would give my right arm if I could have her back with no suffering on her part. My wife was eighty, and I was eighty-five at the time of her death. We were both a-pack-a-day smokers having started the habit in our early twenties. My gripe is that a smoker is not being fair to their family and those who inherit the position of caregiver. Of course, I do not regret one minute spent in giving her my undivided attention. I wish I had her back. In 1983, I was in the hospital with a respiratory problem, and upon discharge, my physician advised that if I stopped smoking I would probably add five years to my life span. I stopped immediately. To date, it has been ten years. I have emphysema. It is not severe; I can do almost anything a person my age is capable of doing. After my return from the hospital, and for several years following, I pleaded, begged, and implored my wife to stop smoking.

This is my gripe: Not being an M.D., my prediction may not hold water; however, I believe that had my spouse quit smoking, she would be alive today.

Currently, my life is lackadaisical and without direction. I have few friends, and they seem to live as couples—not singles. Having my spouse (a common smoker) leave is like having the bottom drop out of my life. It is difficult to understand why people continue to smoke when so much information is available to demonstrate that continuing the practice leads to eventual suicide. Tobacco ruined our lives and took hers—it could have been avoided.

He Wouldn't Accept the Fact That Smoking Was Turning Me Off—A Former Smoker

My husband's smoking has affected our marriage, our children, and me. It hurt our marriage so much that it contributed to our divorce four years ago.

When we were first married in 1966, my husband smoked cigarettes. He said he had started at thirteen. For about the first ten years, it didn't bother me too much, or perhaps I was just willing to put up with it. Then, I got tired of the smell in the house and in the car, in my clothes, and hair. Also, it was pretty expensive, and we just did not have the money to throw away on cigarettes. I begged and harassed him to stop smoking. He switched to the pipe as a compromise and even told me that he had quit. I wondered why he kept taking trips away from the house several times a day when he was home for the weekend, until I found his cigarettes in the car. I was very hurt and felt betrayed because he had hidden it from me. But a part of me also felt like I was being unreasonable to ask him to stop doing something that he enjoyed.

After he switched to the pipe, things became worse. He smelled of smoke all the time and I couldn't stand to be close to him because his breath was so bad. I loved him a lot, and I've always enjoyed physical intimacy, cuddling, and kissing, but even gum didn't help because the smell seemed to be in his lungs. He did not brush his teeth very often, unless he out-and-out had sex on his mind. I couldn't stand to sit next to him in the pew at church because the smell was so bad. The kids would make comments about their father's bad breath. Nothing seemed to faze him. He would ask me why I didn't like to be close to him anymore, and when I told him, he would try gum again, but that was it.

He also had a severe snoring problem. Our physician said it was partly due to the smoking and recommended a sleep clinic. I heard him stop breathing for brief periods of time during the night. He never went to the sleep clinic. During the last five or so years of our marriage, sex or any type of intimacy was a real nightmare. I could not stand to be close to him, but I was willing to have sex just as long as he didn't breathe on me. There was no build-up to sexual enjoyment, because I couldn't stand to kiss him. He would pursue me all the time, I think because sex was not satisfying for him. He wouldn't accept the fact that his smoking turned me off. It was a real vicious cycle. I thought there was something wrong with me. We went to marriage counselors for two years, but he was never willing to do the work that they suggested we do. Of course, there were a lot of other problems in our marriage, but I know if he had not been a smoker, things would have turned out differently.

Smoking also affected his participation in the family. For the last five to eight years of our marriage, he decided to smoke only outside the house and not in the car. That was great; I used to think it a great sacrifice for him. But in reality, it was more of a sacrifice for the children and me. After work and on weekends, he spent the majority of his time at home smoking and reading outside. He was never in the house to deal with the little family upheavals that occur with children from day to day. He was not able to hear their stories and excitement, or to interact with them. He wasn't there to help them or me. When he was inside talking to me, I could tell that his mind was not fully on what we were talking about because he had that inattentive look in his eye. If there was a pause in the conversation, he was outside again. Now our daughters are grown and away from home. They said they would never smoke. Now, they both smoke cigarettes. Both have tried to cut down on smoking but were unsuccessful. Our son stays with his dad on the weekends and the rest of the time with me. He hates going there because of the smoke. His dad smokes indoors and in the car.

My ex-husband's smoking adversely affected our sex life and our communication. I feel very strongly about this, and now that I've been apart from him for four years, I can accept the fact that the problem of his smoking was not something I made out to be bigger than it really was. And, I am still angry! I do not understand how someone who says they love you cannot make more of an effort to change what is destroying your relationship.

I Did This to Myself—A Lifelong Nonsmoker

Dave, my husband, was diagnosed with lung cancer on January 4, 1989. At the time of diagnosis, he was told he had only four to six months to live and that they could offer him radiation and chemotherapy to slow down the cancer and shrink the cancer cells. Dave had started smoking when he was fifteen. His mother had smoked before him. Dave smoked two or more packs a day.

I met him in college, back in those years when the hazards of smoking were not well known. As time went by and the risks of smoking became clearer, I begged him to stop, telling him, "Those cigarettes will kill you." He was totally addicted and only made a few half-hearted attempts to quit. I believe he looked at his mother who smoked and was "healthy" and felt he would be healthy too.

Dave did not feel well for six weeks prior to his diagnosis. He had shoulder pain, bursitis, problems urinating, and was very, very tired. When diagnosed with primary lung cancer he learned it had already spread to the brain, bone, liver, and bladder; it was everywhere.

Dave made two comments after the doctor walked out of his room: "I just received my death sentence," and "I did this to myself." I started crying and Dave told me to leave. He couldn't deal with the diagnosis and me at the same time. He said I had to be strong and I just couldn't at that point.

Our relationship was great. We were best friends for twenty-six years. Dave died when he was only forty-eight. He was an exceptional person: an Eagle Scout; went straight to college after completing the eleventh grade; had degrees in nuclear engineering; attained US patents and papers and the position of vice president of a fortune 500 Company. Most brilliant people are a little one-sided in personality, but not Dave. He was witty, funny, and brilliant. He loved people, and everyone loved him.

We were always able to communicate and would spend hours talking on a Saturday night, if we weren't going out. We'd turn on the stereo and dance in the foyer of our house laughing and talking.

After Dave's diagnosis and with a little time, Dave and I started working as a team. Dave wanted to do everything to extend his life, and we worked together to accomplish this. At the end of the first three months after diagnosis, Dave said, "Let's go for three more months," and we fought for that time. My main goal was to keep him going.

Dave was admitted to the hospital several times, mostly pulmonary related. The one I remember the most vividly was in April; he was admitted because he could not breathe. Dave asked me if he was going to die. He was admitted for the last time in June, and I had to tell him that he wouldn't be coming home again. Dave then made up his mind to end his life as quickly as possible, which wasn't easy because he had an athletic body. At the end, the oncologist and I made the decision to take him off everything but pain medication, and let him go. He died forty-eight hours later in my arms, surrounded by his family.

At the end, I told him I loved him, that I would take care of our children, and that my parents would watch over all of us. I told him that it was okay to leave and to go with God. After he died, we stayed in the room for thirty minutes and we told Dave we loved him; we surrounded his bed; my mother holding one of his hands and I the other, forming a chain. We said the Lord's Prayer and then called the nurse to let her know Dave had died.

One of the mainstays during Dave's illness was family and friends. Not a day went by that we didn't receive phone calls, cards, flowers, gifts, and visits. Dave and I had friends all over the country. Two couples, one from Oklahoma and one from Tennessee, flew in for a weekend during his illness to see us and for his funeral. The outpouring of love was wonderful.

Sarah, our daughter, saw Dave for the last time in March. She was eight-and-a-half months pregnant. Saying goodbye for death was very difficult. She lived in Oklahoma, we in Virginia. She had come up to stay for a month. During that time, she spent as much time as she could with him. She was twenty-four. After Dave's death, she had pictures everywhere and claimed she could smell his cigarette smoke when she went into a room. She then went the opposite way and removed all his pictures. Now, almost five years later, she has a picture of him in her bedroom and can talk easily about him.

Our son Randall was nineteen when Dave died. During Dave's illness, he was very angry with his father for dying and expressed his anger frequently. Dave wanted Randall to go to Texas A&M, and we called admissions in May to find out if Randall had been accepted. We told them his dad wanted to know, and they were kind enough to tell us Randall had been accepted. Dave died in July. Randall went to Texas A&M in August.

For the first year and a half at Texas A&M, Randall told no one that his dad had died. He joined his dad's fraternity, but never told his fraternity brothers that his dad was dead. At Christmas a year and a half later, I gave Randall a framed photograph composite of his dad's fraternity and his pledge certificate. He took those back to school. For the first time, he had a picture of his dad and was able to talk about him and acknowledge he had lost his father. Randall graduated from A&M with a degree in economics and is now a salesman of computer software. He is doing very well. He has a girl he dates, and if things keep progressing, I expect they'll marry within the next year or so.

I have never felt such deep emotional pain as when Dave died. I felt I'd lost part of me. I joined a bereavement group at the hospital for six months, and it was a lifeline for me. I have since remarried and have tried to move forward. As I tell people, when you lose someone you love, you can either lay down and die or get up and go on; going on is a lot harder.

I now work as an administrator at the hospital where Dave died helping families with dying and recently deceased family members. Two years prior to Dave's death, I had lost my thirty-nine-year-old brother in an auto accident, and three years after Dave's death, my other brother died from a hemorrhage.

Our family is unique in that none of my parents' grandchildren have a father. I believe that the grief never leaves you. I don't understand why one family should have so much sadness, because we are a good, decent, and loving family. My only conclusion is that everyone is born with a lifetime, and Dave, Jack, and Allen lived theirs. My life was changed forever by Dave's death. Our dreams died, and new dreams had to replace them. As time goes by, I feel healthier mentally and emotionally. Time is the only thing that really helps, as well as a willingness to let time heal. I rarely go to the cemetery. Dave, Jack, and Allen are buried side-by-side. I don't feel they are there spiritually. They are in the sky, the wind, the beautiful day. There is an underlying sadness to my life and yet also a need to live life fully, to not put things on hold. I truly understand how quickly life can end and how fragile it is. When Dave died, our family unit was destroyed. Our center was gone; the kids and I have flailed about since, trying to find "our family" again.

I have no bitterness. I don't know why I don't, but it's a wasted emotion and only hurts the one who harbors it. Plus, bitterness and anger take a tremendous amount of energy that I'm unwilling to expend.

The tobacco industry gets away with murder, but Dave said, "I did this to myself." He made a very bad choice to smoke, but it was his choice, and it hurt his family deeply. Unfortunately, my story is not unique. Go to any hospice unit in any hospital and you will hear it told over and over again.

It's Me or This—A Lifelong Nonsmoker

I grew up one of nine children in North Carolina. No one in the family smoked in the early years while I was growing up, although some of my older sisters did smoke after they left the home. I had many relatives and do not remember anyone smoking. There might have been some tobacco chewing. I can remember some smoking among girlfriends in high school, and I might have tried it a few times. It looked very glamorous in the movies. Cigarettes were very cheap and advertised heavily: "I'd walk a mile for a Camel," and so on…

I married a man from Newton, Massachusetts, when I was nineteen. He was eleven years my senior and had a career in the military. He smoked. I thought nothing of it. He kept smoking and smoked through three children and thirty years of marriage. We lived in Europe for two different three-year periods. He continued to smoke—probably two packs a day. I remember only one time that he tried to quit: He acted like a zombie and resumed smoking soon after. It was a way of life; he never was without cigarettes, which he bought in advance by the carton. Through the years, he suffered from various stomach problems, sore throat, and other minor physical ailments. He was always cold when I was warm. He had dental problems and eventually lost his upper teeth due to gum problems. Although he was addicted to the cigarettes, he was an intelligent, witty, kind, and generous husband and father. This addiction brought on an early death due to lung cancer at the age of fifty-eight.

When it all began, he was not sick, and he just felt tired. An X-ray showed a spot on his lung so he went into the hospital for a biopsy. The doctors came out of the operating room to tell me that he had cancer and emphysema. If he survived intensive care for three days, he could live six months. He lived seven days.

By the time he died he had virtually no lungs. My son was fourteen, my middle daughter was graduating from high school in a week, and my oldest daughter had been married for a short time. His early death has had a profound effect on their lives. In fact, my son is just now dealing with his grief.

Since his death, I allow no one to smoke in my home. I hate to see friends and coworkers struggle with the problem, so many of them rationalize it away. I see the contrast in my sisters' looks and health when we get together. I can tell the smokers among women my age by the wrinkles and circulation in their hands. I deal with the public in my work, and young girls and women destroy their beauty with smoking every day. The smell of smoke under perfume is sickening. I am appalled by the ads showing healthy, beautiful young people smoking. They should show some of the smokers later, when their looks and health have been ruined. I hate the "You've come a long way baby" advertisement. Ads are definitely aimed at the young. They should not be permitted to glorify smoking the way they do. In the city, there is a VA hospital; it is horrifying to see the cases of smoke-induced problems there.

I remarried after ten years to a man five years younger than me. He used Skoal. I realized this only after we married; he did it so discretely. He liked to say that he quit smoking. I had always been passive and accepted the smoking during my first marriage, but no more. I asked a dentist that we both knew to tell me some things about the effects of the chewing tobacco. He wasn't very talkative, but he came unhinged at my question and launched into a lengthy discussion of the horrors of chewing. I told my husband what he had said, but promised him that I would not nag him about it. He didn't quit. Finally, one day we were talking and I discovered that he had some tobacco in his mouth. I told him that if we were going to live together, I would have to take up the habit, so I put some in my mouth and was so sickened and disgusted I said, "It's me or this!" He quit, cold turkey, and hasn't used it again. It has been six years now. However, for the first six months he had withdrawal symptoms, was irritable, and had numerous aches and pains; further, his libido has never been the same. His lips and hands looked blue a lot of the time, but now he looks healthy.

The tobacco companies are now trying to defend themselves by saying that smoking is a habit, not an addiction. They are wrong-dead wrong. In the flower shop where I work, I help families arranging for flowers to bury their loved ones. I hear heart-breaking stories and see their grief. I have come to hate the "habit" and thank God that I never developed one.

We live in an area in Tennessee where tobacco is grown and subsidized by the government. This is such a paradox now that so many laws are being passed to prevent smoking.

CHAPTER 3

Parent–Child Relationships

For many smokers, the act of smoking is enough to indict them as bad parents, and many recount instances when subjected to the humiliation and abuse of public indictment. It is difficult for smoking parents who must deal with personal pressures to quit as well as the guilt and shame of addiction to be constantly vulnerable to public abuse from strangers. The many defensive accounts in the narratives of smokers of healthy children despite smoking throughout pregnancy and child development speak to the volatility of this issue. While most unrepentant smokers vehemently dispute the notion that smoking adversely affects children, former smokers are generally quick to confess guilt about the effects of their tobacco use on the welfare and health of their children. Many do feel that their smoking is what caused their children to take up the habit.

Many children whose parents and other relatives smoked now smoke as adults. Some point out that their habits began when they were born to smoking parents. Nonsmoking children of smokers describe in detail the effects of their parents' habits on their emotional and physical health through childhood, adolescence, and adulthood. Many complain of constant childhood and continuing chronic battles with asthma, bronchitis, and pneumonia; for these and other reasons, many of these nonsmoking children become estranged from their families. It is clear that some children of smoking parents feel hurt, confused, and angry when

I. Newman and J. DeFrain, *Tobacco Use and Intimate Relationships*,
https://doi.org/10.1007/978-3-319-92579-0_3

their parents deny that secondhand smoke affects them. Many parents, whether consciously or not, worry extensively about their sickly children, but cannot or will not connect their child's illness with their smoking habit. When confronted by children who feel sick and miserable due to smoke, some parents even tell their children that their symptoms are "made up." These and other parents must deal with their guilt every day, acknowledged or unacknowledged.

To complicate matters, it is difficult for smoking parents to discipline their children or advise them against tobacco use for the sake of their own health. Many feel hypocritical about disciplining children when fully aware of their own faults. It is no far reach to infer that this only adds to parental guilt about smoking. Conversely, many smokers recount experiences in childhood and early adolescence when a smoking parent's strict rebuke and nonambivalent stance on smoking might have deterred them from continuing the habit. Many smoking adults express confusion over their parents' ambivalence or silence about the dangers of tobacco and believe that it permitted their early use of the habit-forming substance. Certainly, the smoking parent's own ambivalence about or denial of the dangers of smoking must in part explain this problem. However, this does not stop some smoking parents from refusing to allow their children to smoke, or at least limiting the habit until later adolescence and adulthood. Smoking children of nonsmoking parents may hide their habit for years from their parents.

Many smokers do not believe that smoking affects their families adversely. If smokers do address how smoking affects family dynamics, they almost always deflect responsibility away from themselves, painting unflattering portraits of family members who are intolerant of their desire, need, and right to smoke. Smoking parents, for example, point out the hypocrisy on the part of children or other family members who do not allow smoke around themselves and their children and yet allow their children to visit extensively, knowing that they will be exposed to smoke. A central issue here for smokers is the right to smoke in one's own space—most smokers feel it an invasion and violation of their rights and space when they are asked not to smoke in their own homes, for example. It is clear that parents also feel rejection and humiliation when asked not to smoke in the presence of their children's families or in their homes. For many, as the habit is an integral part of their identity, certainly to reject the behavior is to reject the smoker herself. The silence that surrounds smoking in families is related to intense emotions that tend to inhibit compassion, disclosure, or discussion. These emotions can deteriorate into feelings of resentment and anger, which in turn lead to the estrangement of loved ones. Where communication, empathy, and support are necessary for everyone involved, many parents and their children choose instead to isolate themselves from each other, and many do not see each other at all.

Furthermore (and this affects all members of the family), the time a parent, partner, or other family member spends smoking away from the rest of the family is time that could have been spent with the family. A consequence of this is that some children do question their parent's love and loyalty, believing that their smoking parent's foremost priority and first love is tobacco. It is ironic that a disappearing parent often does so to save their family from the discomfort of secondhand smoke. This division of time between family and habit is particularly difficult for the smoker's spouse and children to accept and, again, must complicate the grief process when such a family member becomes ill or dies because of tobacco use.

Perhaps the most moving accounts of the effects of smoking on families come from smokers and nonsmokers alike dealing with (or for the smoker, perhaps not dealing with) the death of a smoking parent(s), spouse, sibling, or other close relative. For nonsmokers and former smokers dealing with the death of family members caused by heavy smoking, the unresolved emotions that surround smoking in the family complicate and lengthen the process of grief. It is clear that for some smokers—whose disclosures of the deaths of family or intimate friends are invariably obscured by their denial of the link between smoking and illness or death—the premature death of a smoking parent might also be left unresolved and perhaps add to the likelihood of tobacco use and addiction. For nonsmokers, especially if they have become caregivers to loved ones, the silence around smoke-related illness or death is difficult, particularly if other family members continue to smoke and will not acknowledge the role of tobacco in the loved one's illness or death. Unfortunately, for many nonsmoking and smoking children alike, the smoking-related illness or death of a loved one is something they must constantly anticipate and fear.

Testimony

I don't feel like smoking has affected my life or my family one way or another. ***It is the only way my family knows me. They accept it and never say anything about it.*** *(an unrepentant smoker)*

*****

I strongly believe that my addiction to nicotine began at birth. *I believe that I was born with a genetic predisposition to smoke. Both my parents were smokers and my mother was also an alcoholic. All of my uncles and many aunts smoked. My older sisters smoked when they became teenagers. All my parents' friends smoked and as I became a teenager, so did my friends. (a smoker who believes she can't quit)*

*****

I smoked through four pregnancies. Nothing was the matter with any of the kids *and they were all average weight. (an unrepentant smoker)*

*****

When I became pregnant with my second child, for three months I became ill if I smoked or was near smoke. In the fourth or fifth month I was able to smoke again and enjoyed it. Doctors did not warn us against smoking back then. ***It's hard to convince my children not to smoke when I'm still smoking myself.*** *We can't let go of it. My sons both smoke. They do not feel good about it and are feeling the effects. I suppose in a way I taught them to smoke when they were still at home. One was born a premature baby. He has many respiratory problems. My youngest son's smoking also hurts his health. (a mother who believes she can't quit)*

*****

I did not start smoking until after my children were born. I don't think it would have damaged them had I done so. *I think our bodies adjust to whatever environment we grow up in. If they didn't, our species would have died out long ago. (an unrepentant smoker)*

*****

My wife was pregnant with my daughter and I pleaded with her to quit. She said she did, but I caught her sneaking them and it hurt me terribly. (a husband whose wife believes she can't quit)

*****

I taught myself how to smoke at 14. ***I "trained" on my father's Camel non-filter cigarettes.*** *I am currently 42 and smoke three packs of cigarettes a day. (a smoker who can't quit)*

*****

I never encouraged anyone to smoke or not to smoke. *Of our children, the forty-three- and forty-two-year-olds have never smoked. The thirty-three-year-old started last year, the thirty-one-year-old smoked for a year or two near age twenty, the twenty-five-year-old has smoked for the last two or three years and the twenty-four-year-old has never smoked. (an unrepentant smoker)*

*****

You could tell when my husband needed a cigarette: He became frustrated and short-tempered. ***It made us angry that he smoked, because if he was he a victim of tobacco use, so were we!*** *Emotionally it was difficult to have a smoker in the family. My husband only smoked in the garage, and when he came inside the children would tease and scold him. He was sending them mixed messages: Do what I say, not what I do. (a former smoker)*

*****

My husband and I have had six children, each of whom weighed up to nine pounds, ten ounces. None of them have had any lung troubles. (an unrepentant smoker)

*****

We had two girls, thirteen months apart. They are perfectly normal. *One was seven pounds, one ounce and 18 inches long and the second was seven pounds, three ounces and 21 inches long. So much for low birth weights. Both got some college, and the first is an enrolled agent, the second worked as an accountant, later becoming a licensed, bonded livestock buyer and the bookkeeper for her husband's business. So much for brains. (a woman who believes she can't quit)*

*****

I will always deeply regret having smoked. We have six children, four of whom smoked-three of whom still do (one is now frying to quit). ***To have "inspired" your kids to smoke is a rotten legacy.*** *We were not forceful enough talking to our children about smoking, and in most cases were ignored. Now I feel that it's way late, but hopefully not too late to be more vocal and open about my opposition … The old guilt and hypocrisy thing kept me quiet. But now my view is changing. (a former smoker)*

*****

I have sat in a restaurant and gotten looks and comments that would kill because I lit a cigarette after dinner. I don't comment to anyone if they choose not to smoke. I feel like I am looked at like I care nothing for my home, my family, my health or my children. ***I feel I am treated like a contagious leper. The fact is that my home and my family are my top priority. They are my life.*** *(an unrepentant smoker)*

*****

My story begins on December 9, when my second child was born, weighing a healthy nine pounds and five ounces. He was immediately isolated, but no one could figure out what was wrong. One doctor thought it was the flu. At that time there was not much said about smoking while pregnant. My son was in and out of the hospital until he was 12. At age seven they tested him for allergies and found some. He had to have adrenaline many times. ***About three years ago he said to me, "Mom, I think your smoking caused my asthma."*** *I was shocked, but over the years I have had to deal with a great deal of guilt because I have read reports on studies connecting asthma to smoking. Alan is much better now as an adult, but he always carries an inhaler.* ***I am convinced now that my smoking marked him for life. This is hard to live with.*** *(a former smoker)*

*****

I do have a problem with holier-than thou nonsmokers giving me advice on my private life. If someone visits my home, I tell them that if they do not want to smoke, they will have to not smoke outside. ***My eldest sister does not allow smoking in her house. Therefore, neither my parents nor I visit her, and she rarely visits us.*** *(a smoker who believes he can't quit)*

*****

As a college student away from home, I noticed that few of my friends smoked. When I would visit home, the smell was overwhelming. All my things smelled when I returned to campus. ***I attended school only a fourteen-hour drive from home, but I returned less and less frequently.*** *After college and graduate school I got married.* ***My mother is a welcome guest in my home, but her smoking is not.*** *I have three children and a lovely home. She rarely visits. I'm sorry that smoking has come between us. (a nonsmoker)*

*****

How has smoking affected my life? I miss my father deeply—maybe he wouldn't have died so young if he didn't smoke. Maybe my husband wouldn't have had a heart attack, but he's overweight, a couch potato, and drinks and eats the wrong things, so who knows if the smoking is at fault or not. Maybe my bronchitis is made worse—but I had bronchitis before I ever smoked. Other than having a lot more money if we had saved all the money we ever spent on cigarettes, I don't know how else smoking has affected us. ***I feel bad that my kids listened to me preaching about smoking yet have to see me smoke. I feel a little less rejected by them as a result.*** *However, we are a close family so it doesn't really change anything. (a woman who believes she can't quit)*

*****

I grew up in a home where my parents smoked fairly heavily. Back then, in the forties and fifties, I never heard people speak of tobacco smoke being a respiratory irritant, but I knew that I hated tobacco smoke and that it made it hard for me to breathe. I hated the smell of the house when I got home from school every day … My mother always smoked when she was driving. When she would drive me to piano lessons or other places, her smoke would make it hard for me to breathe in the car. ***I asked her once if she would not smoke while I was sitting next to her because it bothered me, and she became angry and said I was making it up.*** *(a nonsmoker)*

*****

I miss my dad a lot [he died of throat cancer caused by smoking]. So do his grandchildren. We just had a large family dinner last evening. ***There was a big hole in the social fabric of our family due to his absence. We all suffer.*** *(a former smoker)*

*****

Smoking makes me feel crazy. There—I said it. And I guess that really is the bottom line. My husband died from cancer eight years ago. For me to smoke in front of my two children is almost unforgivable. They worry (with good reason) that I'll die of cancer. I worry about the second-hand smoke thing, that they'll be more apt to take up smoking themselves. ***Every time I inhale I play these thoughts through my head.*** *(a woman who believes she can't quit)*

*****

There is a glimmer of hope, however. Last week I met with my sister for a few days. We stayed in a nonsmoking hotel and I could only slip out to have my "fix." ***My sister is very special. She never criticizes me although she's never smoked and I know she worries about me, as does my whole family of nonsmokers.*** *Late the last night we were there I excused myself just before bedtime to go downstairs and outside for a cigarette. It was such a major undertaking that by the time I got back up to our room I was ready for another smoke. As I left our room I glanced back at my sister and said something like, "Isn't it terrible?" I saw the look in her eyes as she answered, "I just feel so sorry for you."*

I've thought of that moment ever since and know that somehow I've got to try [to quit] again. ***I can't bear to hurt those I love any longer. Somewhere I must have the strength to walk away from this addiction.*** *(a woman who hopes to quit)*

*****

My first experience with smoking was at an early experimental stage with my brother and friends. ***All our parents smoked; cigarettes were always readily available in fancy cigarette boxes around the house. We would smoke to look, act, and play like grown-ups.*** *(a smoker who can't quit)*

*****

Children raised in smoking environments often suffer mental and physical damage but are often powerless to make changes to their own environments. (a nonsmoker)

*****

I feel I should be able to smoke in my own home without offending guests. They all know I smoke and should respect my right to smoke in my own home. My nonsmoking children accept my smoking, even around my granddaughters. My nonsmoking stepchildren, however, make an issue of it, waving their hands in the air, coughing, and talking about second-hand smoke. You can see what kind of family trouble this could cause. So, against my grain, I don't smoke as much when they're around; I smoke in another room, which makes me very uncomfortable. ***Although I have the self confidence and assertiveness to mind my own business ... I become a timid, self-conscious, feel-bad-about-myself person in these situations.*** *(a smoker who can't quit)*

*****

Stories

I Smoke. It Makes No Sense!—A Smoker Who Can't Quit

Tobacco use has been the subject of my family's dinner conversations quite frequently. I have been a smoker for the past twenty-two years or so, and my husband has smoked for well over thirty-five years. We are the parents of teenagers whom we of course forbid to smoke. We also have a toddler grandchild that lives in our home; we worry about how our smoking affects her. My husband is about to be a fifty-six-year-old dislocated worker, and we worry about how his addiction will affect his ability to find work. We joke that maybe he'll be able to retire on disability. With all the recent changes in the laws about tobacco use in public and in workplaces, we worry about how we will resolve our problems with our addiction. We have tried many times to quit smoking. We have purchased many of the "do-it-yourself" kits, and my husband has even used the patch under the close supervision of our family doctor. Nothing seems to work!

The physical aspects of being a smoker are sometimes uncomfortable and oftentimes bothersome: The smoke on my clothes is embarrassing; the stains on the walls and on our furniture make for extra housework; messy ashtrays are a bother; the wrinkles on my face are irritating; and it is annoying having to always carry cigarettes or have them nearby. The psychological aspects of smoking are much worse: I feel guilty because I am not strong enough to "just say no"; I fear the health problems that will probably come to pass; I feel too strongly about the need to exercise my "right" to smoke; I feel inferior to others because I am a smoker; and I feel guilty for the health problems that I may have caused my children.

There are many times and circumstances when it's difficult to be a smoker. Recently I've noticed that even purchasing cigarettes is becoming harder. My regular grocery stores have locked the cartons of cigarettes up in a cupboard away from the checkstand. So, after shopping for an hour or so and standing in line for way too long, I have to ask for cigarettes. They are rarely smokers and do not understand the significance of getting the right brand. They call a stock clerk to get the cigarettes, and I usually have to request my brand two or three times before I get what I want. Meanwhile, the people in line behind me are becoming frustrated, a small hassle, a major embarrassment. I usually end up apologizing to the cashier for needing to buy the cigarettes. Even running to a quickie mart to buy a pack of cigarettes often turns into an embarrassing situation. The people in line behind me always seem so impatient when the clerk has to take a second look to find my brand and type.

The greatest psychological stress comes when I think of my smoking in relation to my children. Two of my three children have been smokers. As soon as I knew they were smoking, I confronted them. I confronted them separately—different situations with different kids. Each time I really came down hard on them. I should say we did—my husband and I confronted them together. We had to acknowledge that we are sorry and embarrassed that we smoke and that we don't have what it takes to quit, but we will not let them smoke. At one point, we had to threaten to kick one of our daughters out of the house. I'm sure this was hard for them. Right now, I have one seventeen-year-old and two nineteen-year-olds. I believe that the seventeen-year-old will smoke again in the future. Since she had asthma as an infant, she will really have problems if she ever smokes for any length of time.

My smoking also restricts my activities with my children. My seventeen-year-old is in high school and I would like to be an active parent. I do volunteer to do things that I can do at home or that I can do in short time periods at school. For example, I would like to be the parent in charge of the band uniforms. I was asked but I had to decline because I can't be at school any longer than two hours at a time. Of course, I don't admit that to the other parents; I make excuses, just like an alcoholic does. I go and spend an hour or two helping tailor uniforms or passing out fundraising materials, but that's my limit. I would really like to be a chaperone on the band trips, but I couldn't tolerate the lack of nicotine. Several years ago, I accompanied a group of students on a two-hour bus trip. After we arrived at our destination, I excused myself and went around a corner to smoke. When the teacher discovered what I was doing, she had a fit. I won't do that again.

My oldest son was involved in sports. We would go to his games but step out at halftime to have a cigarette. The parents that were taking tickets at the gate always had some smart remarks; we quit going to the games. Track season was just as bad. Our son didn't want his friends and their parents to know that we smoked. We would go to the meets just to watch his events and then leave. Again, I was active in the parent booster group, but only when they had short meetings or activities. When they had meals before the track meets, I would cook the food and deliver it to the school—then leave. I would go back afterward to help clean up. All of that just because I needed a smoke.

Our kids seldom invite other kids to our home unless their parents also smoke. They don't tell us about it, but we can see that they are selective. We seldom invite other kids to go places with us unless we warn them ahead that they have to be willing to tolerate smoke in the car.

We also have found ourselves limiting whom we invite to our house for an evening or a meal. Rather than not smoking, we just don't invite nonsmokers. We have many friends who don't smoke and I find that I never invite them over. If they do just "drop-in," we try to reduce our smoking or make sure we sit in a well-ventilated area. It is always a problem.

My husband has problems on the job. He works in an underground mine, so smoking is not allowed for safety reasons. There's not much of a way to argue with that—he chews when he really needs to. He also eats lots of candy. For the first two hours and the last two hour s of his fourteen-hour shift, he is in the office. Smoking is only allowed in one small area of the building. He adheres to that, but he really hates all the smart-aleck comments from his coworkers. His supervisor is a reformed alcoholic and an ex-smoker, and he never passes up a chance to harass my husband—in a humorous way—or so he says.

Then, there is the medical profession. It is amazing what they can blame on a cigarette. You go to the dentist and hear the condescending, "You're a smoker, I see," and the eye doctors attribute vision problems to smoking. We are contemplating changing our family physician because he relates everything to our smoking. We can't get through an office visit without a "gentle reminder" to quit. Believe me, after I've been sitting in his waiting room for an hour, I don't need to be reminded that I want a smoke.

The hospitals are another big irritant. The no-smoking policies are absolutely out of line. When a smoker is hospitalized, the addiction does not just disappear. It is real. It is physical. It needs to be addressed and dealt with. Recently, one of my husband's coworkers was hurt while at work. He was taken to the hospital and had surgery on his hand. When my husband got off work, he asked me to take the guy a cigarette; he had been in the hospital for ten hours or so and was desperate. I went to the hospital and offered the smoke. Of course, the nurses were not pleased, but the guy wanted it bad enough to get out of bed and go down two floors to the outdoor sitting area—trailing his IV. The medical profession has got to acknowledge smokers' addictions.

Last year, my mother died of cancer in a hospital in Los Angeles. I went to California to be with her and my father through the last four weeks. Mother did not want to be left alone even for one minute, so for many days my dad and I took turns sitting with her for twenty-four hours a day. I had to go outside in order to have a cigarette. It was bad enough having to leave mom alone long enough to satisfy my addiction. Standing outside the hospital in the 110-degree heat was tough. At night, it was awful. Standing around in the dark in a city where crime is rampant was downright terrifying. The doors would lock as I went out, so I'd have to wait for someone to wander by and let me back in the building. During those long night shifts, I could usually go four hours without a smoke break, but I'm sure the whole ordeal could have been much more tolerable if the hospital would have at least provided a secure area for me to smoke. Cheaper, too. Every time I went out someone would come up to me to beg cigarettes and/or money. I was too scared to refuse.

My dad has severe asthma and emphysema. Maybe because he got some kind of lung disease while he was in the Air Force in Europe during World War II and didn't receive appropriate treatment? Maybe because he smoked heavily for more than thirty years? Maybe genetics? His dad died of lung problems, and all four of his brothers suffer from the same problems. Who knows? At any rate, on a bad day he has to use oxygen often. Some days he doesn't need the oxygen, but he uses enough drugs to finance his own pharmacy. It is obviously a problem for him that my husband and I smoke. We break his heart every time we light up. I'm sure he feels guilty that I smoke. He is the only person who makes us not smoke in our own home. It's not that he insists, but we do it out or respect for him. When he comes to visit, we smoke outside. When we go to his house, we smoke outside. A few years ago, we went to a family reunion at his house. We stayed in his RV so that some of the older relatives could be in the house. I smoked a cigarette in his RV one night. I was having intestinal blockages, and the pain was unreal. I didn't have the strength to get up and go outside, but I couldn't sleep and I needed a cigarette. I felt like such a criminal. I was afraid to face my dad for the rest of our stay. I'm sure that he never knew, but I felt absolutely awful. I told my older brother, and I'm sure that he told my dad. To this day, I feel like a little kid waiting to be "called on the carpet."

In just weeks, I am going to Des Moines for a family reunion. My husband and I have decided that we will have to stay in a motel rather than with relatives because of our smoking. Some of these aunts and uncles I haven't seen for thirty years and I will have to limit my time with them because of my ugly habit. What will they think of me? My mother just died of cancer, and my father is disabled with lung problems. I smoke—It makes no sense!

We recently ended our association with our church because of our smoking. Even though we never smoked in the presence of the other church members, we felt that they thought we weren't good enough Christians because we could not give up our habit. Once in a while one of them would ask if we'd made any progress quitting. We just felt like our smoking was getting in the way of our being a part of the church body. Now our kids are deprived of a home church due to our habit. They are old enough to attend on their own, but it has always been a family thing. They lost out again.

I used to have a full-time career for many years as an administrative assistant. I gave it up a couple of years ago because one of my kids needed me to be around full time to keep her from dropping out of high school. Within the next year, we expect to move to Arizona and I hope to resume my career. All the restrictions on smoking in the workplace scare me to death. I seriously don't know how I will be able to go four or eight hours without smoking. At home, I smoke when I use the phone, the computer, and the adding machine. On my last job, I was able to smoke in my own office with the door closed, if the company executives were not in town. If they were around, I had to hide out in the back of the building—outside. I have joked that maybe I will have to go on disability because no employers will hire a smoker. Employers seem more willing to pay for rehab for a drug addict than to tolerate a smoker. I really wonder what the solution will be. Reformers who talk of making tobacco illegal scare me. If they make tobacco illegal, they will make me a criminal.

I don't want the sympathy of nonsmokers. But perhaps I do want their compassion. When they are so busy creating smoking regulations, they need to remember that my smoking is a real physical and emotional addiction. I want the medical world to acknowledge that my addiction is real. I want to be a nonsmoker.

If I Smoke Now, I Die—Plain and Simple—Former Smoker

I have definitely been burned by my habit. I am a thirty-nine-year-old mother of three, and I have smoked since high school. My parents smoked before me, as did theirs before them. Last month I was diagnosed with emphysema. Apparently I have been asthmatic all my life; my smoking masked the symptoms. I have lost thirty percent of my lung capacity, and it is only because of the large tubes in my lungs that I am not dead. The smaller branch tubes and end sacks no longer work, nor will they ever work again.

This was an expensive disease: twenty-five years of smoking, at $4 (Canadian) a day equals $36,500 (Today the price is $13.00 Canadian). Smoking has cheated my family out of all the luxury this money could have bought, plus the probability of their children ever having a grandmother. Tomorrow I see a cardiologist to see how much damage my heart has sustained from this filthy habit. I quit smoking one month ago—the day I was diagnosed.

I began smoking around fourteen when it was cool. It was easy to sneak cigarettes from my mother—she chain-smoked. Both my parents smoked, as did most of my grandparents. I remember my first time in the hospital with pneumonia and pleurisy; I was six. I had numerous encounters with both diseases throughout the years. Later on, I married and had three low-birth-weight babies—I never admitted that smoking could be the cause. I struggled on through life trying to afford the necessities and support my habit—it wasn't easy. I reverted to rolling my own cigarettes to save a bit. I avoided friendships if I couldn't smoke in their homes and other situations where I couldn't smoke. The almighty cigarette ruled my life. I always had a cold, but when I quit now and then for a few months at a time, it would go away. Now it doesn't ever go away.

About four months ago I started running into trouble. My oldest son's eyes were irritated. I took him several times to our doctor for drops, but they stayed the same. In the back of my mind, I knew it was the smoke but I shut it out. One day I had a cold so bad that I could hardly breathe (could still smoke though). I was sent for X-rays, told to rest and come back in a week or two, and told to try to cut back on my smoking. Three days later I was back. I just couldn't breathe at all. My doctor sat me down and bluntly told me that my smoking had caused my babies' low birth weight, my son's eye irritation, my asthma and now-emphysema. I was immediately sent to a respirologist and a cardiologist to monitor my overworked heart. If I smoke now, I die—plain and simple. My kids are paranoid I'll start again. Terrified. I have lost the wonderful voice I used to have. I gained weight each time I quit smoking and have premature wrinkles. And, I have not taught my own kids the value of a healthy lifestyle.

I have been hypnotized, tranquilized, patched, chewed, and layered. I tried acupuncture and cold turkey. Nothing helped till it was too late. I started smoking again every time. I blamed it on the method; it wasn't quite good enough. Finally, the doctor told me to just quit—all by myself. That way I would have nothing or no one to blame but myself. Given the circumstances, so far I'm doing well. I work in the emergency department of a hospital and see emphysema patients come in frequently, pulling along their oxygen bottles, barely alive, merely watching the world go by and no longer participating. It's a pretty scary future to envision.

I Feel Hateful Toward My Mother—Former Smoker

Having a loved one sick and dying from an illness is heart-wrenching. My mother is fifty-nine years old. She smokes at least three packs of cigarettes a day. She has emphysema, Crohn's disease, and often suffers from bouts of pneumonia, bronchitis and serious sinus infections. She cannot walk a quarter mile without tiring dramatically. She is thin, pale, and reeks of tobacco. Her home is yellowed and reeks of the foul odor. She coughs constantly and spits up until she is sick in the mornings.

I have seen her turn from a once beautiful woman into one I can only describe as a hag. She has little energy and must rest periodically. She also suffers from headaches that last from one to three days at a time.

To be honest, it is disgusting and makes me very angry. Over the years it has only gotten worse. She has been in and out of the hospital several times. Her most recent trip was due to a blockage. Crohn's disease was the root cause, but the doctor has told us it gets worse and recurs with continued cigarette smoking.

While in the emergency room, my sister and I saw the X-rays of my mom's lungs. When we asked the doctor about the darkness of the X-rays, he showed us a very small part of her lungs that was not yet destroyed by her smoking. We were horrified.

Her doctor has told her to quit; he has given her gum and the patch. She never used either. The worst part of the whole ordeal is that my mom continues to smoke. She knows the damage that has been done. She knows that her continued smoking makes things worse; yet, she will not quit. When she smokes she seems to relax. She seems to think it's impressive. However, it is just revolting.

I feel hateful toward my mother. Our family consists of three girls and a boy. My brother has asthma, and he lives at home with mom. Needless to say, the smoking makes it hard for him to breathe. One of my sisters has major allergy problems as well. Both my brother and my sister have taken shots. My sister still takes shots; she is thirty-seven. I have allergy problems; however, they are not as severe as my siblings' allergies. Another sister has other medical problems, but they are not known to be smoking related. I have a son who adores his grandmother, but he is not allowed to visit her for long periods of time due to her smoking. When he visits for more than a couple of hours he develops sinus problems. This has been observed over the past four years. My mother does not know this is why he isn't allowed lengthy visits with her.

Maybe I am angry with my mother for not quitting because I did. I started smoking when I was about fifteen. It made me feel old, like an adult. My friends didn't all smoke—only a select few did. I enjoyed the taste, the way it would calm me down. I would still like to enjoy a cigarette, but will never again submit!

I sort of tried to quit when I was nineteen. Due to peer pressure, I did not quit in the end, I did not really want to quit. The most difficult part is wanting to quit. No matter how much I needed to quit I did not for a long time want to quit. You must want to quit to be able to quit.

I quit after nine years of smoking. I quit when I found out I was pregnant. It was only then that I wanted to quit enough to do it, finally. When I craved a cigarette after I delivered my first and only child, I realized I was addicted. I still crave cigarettes. And, that is why I will never smoke another.

The hardest part of watching someone who is sick from tobacco use is not understanding why they don't really want to quit, why they won't try, really try, to quit.

I Do Not Want to Be Part of Her Slow, Painful Death—Former Smoker

I have a seventy-three-year-old mother. She has smoked since she was nineteen. She smokes approximately a pack a day. She says her brand has the lowest nicotine and tar content. My mother has a circulation problem in her legs. She weighs seventy-nine pounds on a good day. She also has congestive heart failure; she takes fourteen pills a day to keep her heart going and her fluids down. Because of the circulation problem in her legs, she can barely stand for more than five minutes and can only walk short (very short) distances with a cane or supported by a shopping cart.

She can drive but just can't walk. I do all of her errands, from taking out the trash to purchasing groceries, medicine … I have made such a fuss about her smoking that I will not purchase cigarettes for her. For that, she gets in the car and goes to the 7-11.

Two years ago she was hospitalized for twelve days with a heart problem. When I went to pick her up, she had called the hospital gift shop to ask them if they sold cigarettes and would deliver some to her. Once I got her home, she called her apartment maintenance man and paid him twenty dollars to go out in the snow and buy her a carton of cigarettes.

Her doctors say the smoking is not good for her health and have encouraged her to try to quit; they all suggest that it is hurting her walking. However, with each examination (every five months or so) her lungs are clear. She takes that to be okay to smoke. She's had six doctors and no doctor will ever be firm and tell her to quit. I have privately asked them to do this in confidential letters. Still, no one tells her to quit.

She derives great pleasure from smoking. She has little to do but read, watch TV, sleep, eat and smoke. I have to almost force her to go out. I rent a wheelchair and we shop and go to shows and simply picnic, when I can convince her to go out. I have to sit and watch her smoke after each meal and event.

She won't smoke in my car or house. She's a very tidy smoker, never leaving ashes or butts, and she will never smoke in other people's homes. In restaurants, we sit in the smoking area.

So, I know I am watching her die. I have read and looked for explicit information on lung cancer. I do not want to be part of her slow, painful death from cigarettes. I don't want to be around when the doctor says she must have one or both of her legs amputated because of the lack of circulation and the constricted veins.

But what can I do? Nagging does not help. Begging does not help. Being in the hospital, in the CCU and ICU does not scare her enough to quit.

I can only relate to this habit because I love potato chips, Coke and licorice. It would be difficult for me to give these up. Yet I know this is not the addictive habit she experiences. Therefore, I have almost given up with her smoking and have turned to praying for a swift and gentle death when it is her time to go.

My thirty-three-year-old brother sees mother's point of view. He lives in Seattle and visits her about three times a year. While he doesn't encourage her to smoke, he will buy her cigarettes and park her wheelchair where she can smoke. We don't argue; the fact is that I see smoking one way and he sees it another. He doesn't smoke. In fact, all four of mother's children do not smoke. He has told me I should ignore the situation; however, he is not here on a daily basis to see what smoking is doing to her.

I purchase clothes for mother and take them over for her to try on. She can't walk into stores well and it takes a lot of time with her wheelchair. When she decides she doesn't want an item, I must take it home and air it out before I can return it. The entire process of smoking is disgusting.

Sometimes I think this is my problem. She may never die from smoking. I feel selfish that I want her to quit, partially because I don't want the burden of what will happen if she actually dies from smoking. I realize that only time will tell. However, I will never give into her smoking. Every chance I get I encourage my middle school students not to smoke. They are eleven, twelve and thirteen—at a very impressionable age. As a teacher, I know they must be shown what happens when you smoke, not just told.

When the caning incidence happened in Singapore in 1995 my class watched the news channel each day. Almost all twenty-two of my homeroom students voted that Michael should be caned for vandalism. However, one picture made a great impression; when they saw a martial arts person caning a punching bag, they all changed their minds! It was too harsh. This is how smoking education needs to be taught. We have become such a visual society that the students need to see what happens: actual discolored lungs and the pain people suffer.

In my classes, several students want their parents to quit, but a twelve-year-old cannot change an adult.

The hardest part of watching someone who is sick or dying from tobacco is believing them selfish; it may seem that they give little consideration to those who will eventually care for them. I will go through the inconvenience of caring for my mother: shopping, cooking, trips to the hospital. I will experience the pain of her death; she can help, but won't. The thought processes and rituals around explaining scientific knowledge concerning the hazards of smoking fall on deaf ears. The more you nag the more she rebels.

CHAPTER 4

Anger, Silence, and Secrecy

Silence, or perhaps more accurately, secrecy, is an integral part of any addiction. The very complex issues and emotions on "either side" of the tobacco issue unfortunately often disintegrate into a volatile, angry discussion of rights and choice, discourses that do not take into account the intricacies of the issues at hand. For example, when a nonsmoking child asks her smoking parent not to smoke in her presence, or in the presence of grandchildren, often the feelings of either party go undisclosed, and the discussion is simplified down to naked territorial rights. For the smoking parent, rejection of his smoking and denial of his right to smoke threatens his parental rights and authority, which makes him feel humiliated and hurt—like a child. The nonsmoking child's own fear for her parent's health as well as the health of her own family becomes reduced to an expansion of her authority as an adult and parent in her own right. Inevitably, these arguments veil the real emotions of insecurity, humiliation, and fear that both parents and child feel. These genuine feelings are masked by anger, silence, and ultimately, secrecy. The consequence of silence on occasions like these is the deliberate estrangement of family ties, unresolved and continued emotional pain. Certainly, these silences do not help the tobacco addict quit or the nonsmoker find ways to reconcile.

On the part of unrepentant smokers, silences are especially evident in the abruptness of their narratives as well as their narrative forms—fragments of experiences, accounts of abuse, and explosions of anger

I. Newman and J. DeFrain, *Tobacco Use and Intimate Relationships*,
https://doi.org/10.1007/978-3-319-92579-0_4

and hurt. The silences surrounding addiction are evident in the strong defensive tones that their narratives take: “I am healthy,” “My children are healthy,” “Smoking is not an addiction,” and so on. These denials of mainstream opinion and scientific thought sometimes constitute entire narratives. These narratives are extensive and complex. Silences are also evident in the gaps within their narratives as well as the fact that the narratives of most unrepentant smokers tend to be self-focused. It is difficult when one is in denial about a habit to talk extensively about how it affects one’s life, and especially the lives of loved ones.

Unrepentant smokers acknowledge readily that their parents and/or other family members smoked, but most do not go on to say how this affected their lives. In fact, if smokers do confess that a parent or family member died of an illness related to smoking, they do not dwell on the experience at all. This effectively erases the death from their narratives in an act of denial. On the other hand, former smokers and nonsmokers talk exhaustively and in detail about the illnesses and deaths of their family members or friends due to smoking, and it is essential to many of them that smoking is publicly acknowledged as the cause of illness and death.

All the groups of people participating in this project—unrepentant smokers, smokers who wanted to quit but felt they couldn’t, smokers who had quit, and lifelong nonsmokers—included accounts of secrecy in their narratives, specifically that of “closet smoking.” This element of silence and secrecy is a familiar one in many addictions: the veiling of behavior that is publicly censured and indicted, in particular, by ones close to you. For many, this silence is compounded by feelings of guilt and failure, as well as the internalization of much public opinion surrounding addiction: that is, that they are weak- willed, “childish,” and ignorant. For the most part, such secrecy, and the guilt surrounding “closet smoking,” appears only to increase the likelihood of prolonged tobacco use and greater tension within families and partnerships.

Interestingly, one lifelong nonsmoker invokes the rhetoric of the AIDS movement, writing that where tobacco is concerned, “Silence = Death.” It is, thus, everyone’s obligation to speak up against smoking and help educate the community about its dangers.

Testimony

The feeling of uselessness and helplessness was terrible; I simply watched my mother get sick and die. ***I knew if I said anything about her smoking her reaction would just hurt my feelings.*** *(a smoker who can't quit)*

*****

Both my parents tried to quit smoking many times over the years. After my mother was in the hospital, all hooked up to oxygen, she came home and both my parents quit (or so we thought). Each one was sneaking around, trying not to let the other know they were smoking. Then they gave up, went back to smoking openly and were smoking as much as before! (a former smoker)

*****

My boyfriend, Bill, now my husband, had never smoked, and cigarettes repulsed him … [we broke up and] got back together six months later. I didn't tell him I was smoking again. ***Keeping it secret was very stressful—I would try and find every excuse I could think of to go and have a cigarette.*** *Not long after we got back together I became pregnant with my second child. I then quit smoking again, this time for the baby. It was about six months after my son was born that I began smoking again. Bill and I married about a year later. It was sometime after our wedding that Bill found out my smoking secret. It was quite a shock for him; he had no idea I was smoking. It caused some friction in our marriage, but I never smoked in front of him or the kids. I became pregnant again two years later and quit again. Again, after my daughter was born I started smoking. Bill was constantly harassing me, and I demanded he lay off.* ***I felt I was an adult and it was my choice to smoke****, it was also my choice when to quit. Instead of trying to find excuses to go and have a cigarette, I could now smoke outside my house, and in the winter, in the basement. I still did not smoke in front of my husband or children. (a former smoker)*

*****

One of my aunts died of lung cancer, about twenty-five years ago. She did smoke, but ***no one said smoking was the reason.*** *(a smoker who can't quit)*

*****

My brother claims that my father had a "lung cancer gene" that caused him to smoke and made him predisposed to the disease. Anything to avoid the truth, I guess. (a lifelong nonsmoker)

*****

My brother died of lung cancer. When he lost a lung, his doctor told him to quit or he would die; he had been smoking three to four packs a day. He quit and lived ten years, then got lung cancer. He suffered terribly for a year before he died. ***To this day, ten years later, my sister-in-law insists he died from "something in the air" and will not admit that smoking caused his death,*** *although she never smoked and hates smoking. Her sister still smokes at seventy. She admits she is hooked and cannot quit although her daughter (age forty) just quit after a long, hard struggle. Her son still smokes. (a lifelong nonsmoker)*

*****

I found I didn't like sneaking around, but even in later years I lied about my smoking. *When I married, I promised my husband that I would quit smoking. He disapproved of smoking. However, I never did quit. When we divorced, he was the one who spilled the beans and told my family I smoked. I knew my parents would disapprove if they ever found out, especially since my mother was a nurse and had warned me of the side effects of smoking. (a former smoker)*

*****

Talking to our children was not forceful enough. and in most cases, they ignored us. I feel that it's way late now, but hopefully not too late to be more vocal and open about my opposition. However, I find it difficult to admonish our children and even a grandchild who we caught smoking at thirteen—a twinge of hypocrisy hits me, I guess. I tried singing a song I heard some twenty-five to thirty years ago to my grandchild: "Puff, puff, puff that cigarette … Puff, puff, puff it till you're almost dead" (or words to that effect). The finale was a true analysis of the smoker: "…a fire on one end and a fool on the other." The reaction to my singing was a look that said, "There he goes again. " I failed this time, but I will keep trying. ***The old guilt and hypocrisy thing kept me quiet. Now my view is changing.*** *I think our thirteen-year-old grandchild blew my objections away, but that's a poor excuse for silence. Another side effect of tobacco addiction is stealth. Like others I knew who tried to quit, I found myself becoming sneaky. We became closet dwellers, an introduction to a negative lifestyle. (a former smoker)*

*****

The silence has often been deafening. In the presence of a smoker, it is difficult for me to stay and reason because to do so means inhaling their deadly exhaust. Many people seem to feel—and the tobacco industry continues to reinforce the notion—that smokers have a right to do their thing anywhere they please and that those who object to inhaling smoke are just fussy. I've been told

I should just stay home if I don't like it; an addicted surgeon told me that when I asked him to help clear the smoke-filled air at the local hospital. Even those who sympathize are reluctant to speak up when asked if they want smoking or nonsmoking seating at restaurants, often saying it doesn't matter. That is not supportive or helpful. Some who have benefitted from my efforts even tell me that I should remember to be nice about it, inferring somehow that assertiveness and effectiveness are "not nice, not ladylike." This hurts, but silence never got me anywhere; people just seem to want to kill the messenger or anyone who rocks the boat. (a lifelong nonsmoker)

*****

Stories

I Have a Serious Addiction—An Unrepentant Smoker

What is moving about this narrative and many like it is all that is left unwritten. Because it begins with an account of the author's father's addiction to smoking and death, it is clear that this is an important part of the writer's self-concept, and central to understanding his own addiction. However, as is clear from the acknowledgment of his own family's response to smoking, these are issues that the author is perhaps not necessarily ready to integrate and reconcile. Similarly indicative of both the author's acknowledgment and yet tangible silence around the effects of tobacco use and addiction on the family is that he begins and ends his story with incomplete fragments telling of the impact of tobacco use on his family and himself. It is one of the few narratives written by unrepentant smokers that attempts to speak to the influence of tobacco use on loved ones.

I cannot remember a time when my father did not smoke. He never smoked cigars or a pipe. I think he started before cigarettes were on the market. He always, until death, rolled his own. He died of cancer of the stomach when I was thirty-five.

I began smoking cigarettes with any frequency—half a pack per day—when I entered the US Marine Corps at nineteen. The vast majority of my service friends also smoked cigarettes. At twenty-six I became actively involved in my own business. As that business grew, so did my daily consumption of cigarettes until I was smoking nearly three packs a day at the peak of my career. A couple years after my retirement, I was down to under two packs a day. I have been up and down since that time and now, over age seventy, I smoke less than a pack a day.

During my heavier smoking years I tried all kinds of rationing schemes, cessation programs as well as hypnotism, but during none of these attempts to quit did I really want to stop smoking. I went to these ends because from time to time I felt my energy level lacking and felt it could well be from excessive smoking. At age sixty, I had a mild stroke and have since been medicated with blood thinner. I have monthly medical checks.

My wife and three children have been strongly opposed to my smoking for several years and I have not smoked in the presence of my children for at least the past five years. I continue to smoke in the presence of my wife, over her objections and constant reminders that it is extremely detrimental to my health. Obviously, I recognize that I have a serious addiction.

It's So Unhealthy and I Want Him to Live—A Lifelong Nonsmoker

Our family consists of Jack, fifty-two; myself, fifty-one; Philip, twenty-five and Thomas and Allan, both twenty-two. Jack and I have been married twenty-seven years. We met each other in high school; we were neighbors. I've never smoked, and to my knowledge, neither have my children. (Thomas did try chewing for a year or so.) Jack is "our problem."

When we were dating his folks got him a watch for college graduation as a reward for not smoking or drinking. We knew he didn't deserve it. When we got married, I thought he had given up smoking. Over the next ten to fifteen years I'd get clues that he occasionally smoked. People from work would make comments, not realizing I didn't know he smoked. When I confronted him about it he'd deny it. Obviously, he wasn't smoking at home.

In the eighties, he sort of came "out of the closet" about his smoking, but I said absolutely not in or by the house. That meant he would have to go out in the yard. We lived in Austria in the eighties and while there I got an idea to offer to buy him a Mercedes if he stopped smoking. I said I'd take his word for it. In about 1983 he came to me and said, "I'm ready to get the Mercedes. I'm not smoking." He got the car. All was well I thought. Then, once again, people from work would make innocent comments that led me to believe he was smoking. I asked him and he said, "No." I trusted him and believed he was telling the truth. People made more comments—I asked, he denied. Finally, he acknowledged he was smoking some, and the "battle" has been going on since. He pretends he doesn't smoke until irrefutable evidence says otherwise. When he does it's always away from home. When we left Austria we sold the Mercedes because it was too expensive to convert to US standards.

THE BIGGEST PROBLEM: I don't think I'll ever trust him completely anymore. Honesty is the virtue I admire most in life. The Mercedes was a symbol of absolute trust.

When we moved to Duluth, Minnesota, he again declared he wasn't smoking. I again trusted that he was telling the truth. Well, one day I went to his office to pick up something and found him smoking in the break room. It was like catching a kid with his hand in the cookie jar. My heart sank. On one other occasion, I quite by chance drove by him downtown en route to the city hall. He was puffing away on a cigarette but jerked his hand down when he saw me. Again my heart sank.

How did I handle this? Early in the game I politely asked him not to smoke, citing all the reasons why he should quit. On a few occasions, I've offered incentives—the Mercedes was the biggest. Most of the time, right or wrong—probably wrong—I ride him. I criticize him. I give him the cold shoulder. I argue; it's very negative. I am so anti-smoking. It's unhealthy and I want him to live. It's filthy; it stinks and is unattractive. And, last but not least, I don't need to be exposed to it. I'm a big believer in individual freedoms, but not when they infringe on the rights of others. I have the right to clean air in my lungs.

Socially, it is a problem because I am miserable around smoke. We had clear friends in Austria with whom we loved to play Scrabble and other board games. We'd often combine our board games with a pleasant evening meal. Unfortunately, as much as I enjoyed our friends, it's miserable to sit across the table from a chain-smoker for hours—I'd find my lungs screaming for fresh air.

How has Jack's smoking negatively affected the family? In my relationship with him there has been a loss of trust (THE BIGGIE); lack of desire for intimacy when he smells of cigarette smoke and, he denies it but he's irritable because he's constantly experiencing withdrawal symptoms when he can't smoke. Jack has an occasional irregular heartbeat. It blows my mind that he doesn't take every step possible to prevent this condition although it does frighten him.

Actually, I Loved Every Aspect of Smoking—A Former Smoker

Smoking has played a significant role in my life and in the lives of my family members. Both my parents smoked. My mother had an alcohol problem, which when combined with smoking, resulted in her death and a family crisis. She was smoking when she passed out and caused a fire that took her life and everything we had. After this, my father quit drinking and smoking. Of the five of us children, three secretly smoked when my mother died. All but one of us tried tobacco and now only two of us still smoke.

I smoked. Health problems never seemed a threat to me although heart disease is common in my family. My father had heart disease, as did one of his sisters; she had a heart attack at forty. My father died at seventy-three of heart failure. He had two surgeries but lived a full and active life. His sister still smokes, as does his brother. Both have difficulty breathing but seem unconcerned about their health. One of his sisters quit to avoid health problems; she used the patch to help her quit. I quit mainly for social reasons. I quit cold turkey with a friend; the buddy system is good.

When I was growing up my peers didn't smoke; it was seen as crude and unacceptable. I took puffs at a very early age and did my smoking during my teen years. In college, I smoked mainly with my friends. I never smoked in front of my parents.

I loved every aspect of smoking. Before quitting for the last time, however, I had stopped many times for days, weeks, and even months. I promised to quit in my senior year in college because my boyfriend asked me to, but I never did. This short-term quitting was so easy that I would always start back. I smoked in secret much of the time; it was like a premeditated habit. I didn't smoke more than ten cigarettes a day. I enjoyed smoking; I planned activities around it so that I didn't have to smoke in public.

I realized that I was addicted in 1987 and I pledged to my husband that I would quit for good. A friend and I challenged each other (we are both very competitive) to quit. Neither of us wanted to give in; we were good support for each other. I had physical and psychological withdrawal: stomachaches, headaches, irritability, nervousness, depression, and a sense of loss. However, I never did gain weight.

Smoking is "out" in my social circle, but I still allow friends and family to smoke in my home. My family members respect that I don't smoke anymore, and they smoke outside. I wish they would invent a harmless cigarette so I could have all the good without the bad.

I've Always Enjoyed Smoking and Could Stop If I Wished to—An Unrepentant Smoker

I started smoking at sixteen and am still enjoying it at seventy-four. I started by imitating my friends. I have never missed a day of work, rarely have colds and have only been in the hospital twice: forty years ago for a hernia and twenty-five years ago for pancreatitis. I am a fairly active person, taking care of my own lawn work, painting, car washing, etc. I play golf and swim. We have three healthy children and three healthy grandchildren. I do cut down my consumption in the presence of my grandchildren. I spent three years as a navy pilot at a time when cigarettes were free.

One of my aunts died of lung cancer, about twenty-five years ago. She did smoke, but no one said smoking was the reason. My father died of lung cancer in 1936 at the age of forty-seven. He never smoked cigarettes, but on rare occasions, he smoked a pipe.

My only complaint is the expense, but we can handle that. I lately developed a slight cough since I started buying generic cigarettes. I have always enjoyed smoking and still do. I feel I could stop if I wished to.

My wife, also seventy-four, has been smoking since before we were married and has a similar story.

Smoking Is More Enjoyable Than Eating—An Unrepentant Smoker

I had a husband die of lung cancer at thirty-five. I smoke and am concerned about the inaccurate reporting being done about tobacco use.

No one seems to recall that the majority of adults smoked years ago and it has not caused a large number of deaths from lung cancer in our children. Most of us smoked from the time our children were infants. I did and my children are very healthy. If you listened to the hysteria and believed it, a lot of this generation should be dead.

I want to see a report that considers all aspects of this problem. I especially want to know how many died of cancer in the generation that I discussed above. I would hope that this would be interpreted without bias, but in this day that would be unlikely.

I am probably not as upset over all the stigma on smokers because I spend a lot of time at home and am not bothered by other people. I don't mind not being able to smoke in stores, but I don't patronize non-smoking restaurants, except for fast-food places.

We should not be expected to pay more in taxes. There are many reasons why people get sick or die and use a lot of health care besides smoking. The government interferes in too many areas of our life. We are aware of the risks of smoking. If they must interfere, I would prefer them only to have tobacco companies advertise truthfully about the amount of tar and nicotine in their cigarettes. We own a business and I do not believe the government has the right to tell us if we can smoke there or not; we would ignore such a law if enacted.

I started smoking when I was seventeen. All of my friends and relatives smoked. No one worried about health problems in the late fifties. The first cigarettes made me sick so I don't know why I continued to smoke, except that everyone else did and we really did not know the dangers.

My first husband died of lung cancer at thirty-five. He was predisposed to cancer; his father died of cancer and his mother was treated for cancer. His brother died at twelve. He also worked in radar while in the military. I think genetics plays a large part in our health.

My present husband smokes. My best friend has never smoked and she would like me to quit for the sake of my health. It is ironic that she has never smoked and has one health problem after another. I don't have any health problems.

She is genetically predisposed to high cholesterol and has not been careful with her diet. She craves sweets. She has had to try and control it since developing heart trouble, but has trouble quitting in the same way a smoker does. I have doubts listening to her because I have enjoyed good health and am now fifty-six and have smoked quite a few years.

My other friend has been warned for over a year to quit smoking and couldn't do it. She recently had to have a bypass and isn't smoking now, but I'm not sure what will happen when she is feeling better. She also had a very poor diet, which I feel contributed to her problem.

I've tried to quit. I spent $300 on a stop-smoking class but really didn't want to quit and didn't. I tried the gum and that didn't work. Hypnosis worked—I didn't smoke for ten days and didn't want a cigarette. I resumed smoking when I found my daughter murdered by her boyfriend. My attitude toward giving up smoking because of health warnings changed, and I didn't care anymore. I still feel this way, although she died four years ago. When you are going to die is beyond your control, anyway.

When I did quit there were withdrawal symptoms, which were very difficult. I enjoy smoking and don't want to quit; cigarettes have been a part of my life for a long time. Smoking is relaxing—it's more enjoyable than eating. I also find that people who smoke seem to be more sociable and friendly.

I would like to be able to cut down on the amount I smoke, but haven't even done that. I think it is a habit. I am not sure about addiction. I am not as concerned about dying as I am of being old and sick.

If a Person Believes a Behavior Is Harmful Then That Possibility Exists—An Unrepentant Smoker

I have enjoyed smoking for many years and have never considered it an addiction. This may not be true for other smokers. I believe that if a person believes a practice to be harmful to him then that possibility exists. With the hammering that the public gets from all sides on all matters of health, it is a great battle to stay healthy. With the wide dissemination of anti-tobacco information, I'm surprised that tobacco advertising is effective.

I began smoking in high school because friends who smoked seemed to enjoy it. After ten years, I changed to cigars, and fifteen years later changed to a pipe. Changing from cigarettes to cigars to a pipe was not an attempt to quit or reduce smoking.

I am healthy now. Any difficulties that I have are from the battering of my frame, which is still up and going. I think that it is extreme to say that so many diseases are caused by the use of tobacco. To me, a tobacco-caused illness is an uncertainty. To me, smoking is not an addiction. Since we are all psychologically different I realize that to some people the use of tobacco may be an addiction. I am opposed to the US government's use of power more than persuasion to deal with cigarettes.

CHAPTER 5

Personal Rights and the American Way

On both sides of the issue, smokers and nonsmokers alike believe that they have inviolable rights and many invoke the rhetoric of the Civil Rights Movement and American Independence in their narratives. Unfortunately, like many American debates surrounding the contentious issue of choice, neither side of the issue appears to be able to listen to or understand the other. Unrepentant smokers believe that nonsmokers are intolerant and hostile for no particular reason, that they are a privileged majority.

Because smokers for the most part surround themselves with smokers rather than nonsmokers, and because the issue is often wrapped in deadening and tangible silence within families due to the tension surrounding it, many smokers do not believe that secondhand smoke poses a significant health risk to the nonsmoker. This disbelief is very probably exacerbated by the smoker's own denial of the problems of tobacco use to herself and inability to properly acknowledge the effects of her behavior on loved ones, children in particular.

A central issue for many involved is the concept of public and private space. Cigarette smoke, of course, transgresses smoking and nonsmoking boundaries, a fact inescapable for nonsmokers with severe allergies and respiratory ailments, and a fact that seems to evade many smokers. (In all fairness, it is difficult to distinguish the effects of smoke when you are saturated with it from regular and lifelong smoking, and when you do not personally believe it to be harmful.)

I. Newman and J. DeFrain, *Tobacco Use and Intimate Relationships*,
https://doi.org/10.1007/978-3-319-92579-0_5

Choice is inherent to autonomy. The adult smokers who are denied their right to smoke often feel like they are being treated like children—a humiliating experience and one that usually does not lead to reconciliation. On the other hand, nonsmokers hold to their right not to be exposed to smoke. So, is there a compromise to be found? It is clear from all of the narratives that hypocrisy on the part of the government is partially to blame. Nonsmokers would like the government to take a clear and resolute stance on tobacco use. Smokers commonly feel that the government increasingly infringes on their civil rights while profiting from tobacco use. Furthermore, many smokers feel strongly that the anti-smoking movement is biased. After all, many products endanger the health of users and those surrounding them, such as alcohol or fatty foods. They believe that it is hypocritical of the government and mainstream society to restrict their rights, yet not treat alcoholism or obesity as equal issues. Obviously, this imbalance needs to be addressed. For the smoker, the discrimination and persecution is real.

While many former smokers constitute a middle ground in this issue, in that they are able to understand and sympathize with both perspectives—particularly if they suffer from allergies and respiratory problems from smoking—many become themselves intolerant of smoke, becoming what the smoker calls "the born again nonsmoker." For this particular group, and for the majority of lifelong nonsmokers, the effects of secondhand smoke are real and devastating. These populations together tend, for the most part, to see smokers as an indistinct, homogenous group of hostile, inconsiderate, and privileged people—a perspective that smokers also hold to be true of nonsmokers. The perception of privilege is an important one. As smokers' rights become more and more restricted and nonsmokers increasingly feel they have the right to publicly confront smokers, the ritual of confrontation becomes a problematic enactment of power. However, for nonsmokers, especially those with severe respiratory ailments and other allergies, consistent exposure to smoke is a constant reminder of the power of smokers over their lives, health, and livelihood. No party around the issue of smoking can truly be said to have privilege, and the abuse of power only hurts all involved. Again, clearly what is missing is communication, understanding and support, and genuine civility.

Testimony

Smokers with their fatalistic attitudes will say, "You're going to die someday anyway." ***But why do they get to choose how I die?*** *(a lifelong nonsmoker)*

*****

I just finished teaching a unit on Colonial America. ***It is ironic to think that our country was basically founded on the cash crop of tobacco****, among other things of course. If we only knew then. (a smoker who believes she can't quit)*

*****

So what if people smoke? Everyone's tastes are different. Perhaps you don't like the tastes of other people, but individual adults are entitled to their rights. I think people who ask you to not smoke in their presence are overreacting, weak, and angry people. They make me aware of my territorial rights. (a former smoker)

*****

When people ask me to not smoke in their presence my first reaction is anger. After I get past the anger, I feel like they must think I'm inferior, that I am not as good a person as they are because I smoke. I leave immediately to avoid hurting anyone's feelings because of my anger. Of course all these feelings make me want a cigarette even more. Ultimately I would like to be a nonsmoker. But for the time being, I would like to be the one to ask the other person to leave. (a smoker who can't quit)

*****

Most public places provide ample opportunity for conflicts with smokers, and those in authority are often too timid or lacking in motivation to keep a space smoke-free. I can't blame them; ***challenging a person's right to smoke is always like setting off an emotional firebomb.*** *(a lifelong nonsmoker)*

*****

It seems that over the last few years I have fewer and fewer rights. Nonsmokers are constantly complaining about secondhand smoke. I wonder if they have ever been in the same room with smokers who have not been able to smoke for a few hours. Which would be more detrimental to their health, the deprived smokers or the second-hand smoke? ***I am angry that smokers are blamed for***

***anything and everything**: An unexplained fire? Obviously a careless smoker. You catch a cold? You have been around too much second-hand smoke. Never mind that it' flu season and you've kissed everyone in a one-mile radius. If you have a stressful day, you smoke too much. I have sat in restaurants and gotten looks and comments that would kill because I lit a cigarette after dinner. I don't comment to anyone if they choose not to smoke. I feel I am looked at like I care nothing for my home, my family, my health or my children. I am treated like a contagious leper. The fact is that my home and family are my top priority. They are my life. Many years ago in Salt Lake City, Utah I was asked to leave a public restaurant for lighting a cigarette. I was so mad. My money is just as good as anyone else's! Yet I had to leave because I lit a cigarette. I was having some coffee once at an outside cafe when my oldest child was a toddler. She reached for my lighter and I scolded her. A woman at the next table told me if I didn't have to smoke my child wouldn't accidentally burn herself playing with my lighter. I suppose I should also get rid of my kitchen stove so she couldn't burn herself on that either. I told the woman that, and the indignant look on her face was hilarious—I felt very justified in saying it and meant for her to know it. (an unrepentant smoker)*

*****

*When I ask smokers not to light up, just about everyone is cooperative, but some people have an attitude. **I find that most (though not all) smokers are pretty selfish people.** (a former smoker)*

*****

***In today's society it seems as if smokers have no rights and nonsmokers have all the rights.** As I said, next month I am trying out the patch. Hopefully I will become a nonsmoker, with all the rights that entails. (a smoker who can't quit)*

*****

***The anti-smoking movement is filled with misinformation, bias and outright hate. Smokers are made to feel unintelligent and ignorant.** I feel somewhat ambivalent about regulations restricting smoking to certain areas. If all smokers exercised courtesy, it would not be necessary. However, the government (local, state, and federal) has gone overboard, put some businesses out of business, and deprived people of their livelihoods by over-regulation. In our small area alone, the bowling alley has closed, several restaurants have folded, and there has been a rise in unemployment among service-industry personnel due to legislated restrictions. I think it should be up to the business owners. Nonsmokers have a right to choose not to patronize establishments that they feel jeopardize their health or offend their sensibilities. Accommodation should* *be the guideline. In restaurants we are frequently seated in the smoking section only to be accosted by nonsmokers in the nonsmoking section right next to us, or actually in the smoking section complaining about smoke. We are known to quite a few of the restaurateurs, and I have told them, politely, that unless we can be guaranteed a table in the smoking section and that we will not be abused by nonsmokers, we will take our business elsewhere. When we go into restaurants that are nonsmoking, I state loudly and clearly that we refuse to patronize nonsmoking establishments and leave. (a smoker who can't quit)*

*****

***Smoking is an individual's** choice. I have always believed and practiced tolerance; I am no one's judge. We live in a free society. I resent legislation against tobacco products. I had much rather see a tobacco advertisement than a sex-related advertisement. I am tolerant and respect the rights of mankind. (a smoker who can't quit)*

*****

I don't have too many problems with smoke-free zones—if it says "no smoking" then I don't smoke. However, I do feel places of employment should have a designated area where employees can smoke. Our hospital is a very good example: there are people smoking at every entrance, and the butts are an unsightly mess. Wouldn't it be better to have a room with outside vents and control the smoking? (a smoker who can't quit)

*****

***My viewpoint is fairly mixed. I despise smoking, but I do understand that there are people who will fight for their right to inhale dirty chemicals. It is equally the right of nonsmokers to be free of smoke in public.** I resent it when I am in a public place and smoke is blown into my face. Once, at the Schubert Theater in Chicago, a woman got mad at me because my child took a bathroom stall before her, and she blew smoke directly into my face—I am not kidding! (a former smoker)*

*****

*Now at thirty-nine I can't tolerate cigarette smoke at all. I choke up and can't breathe even when someone lights up in the same restaurant. Then my sinus problems act up almost immediately; whenever I'm subjected to smoke I have sinus problems and get a terrible sinus headache. **Some people think it's silly and ridiculous to make a fuss over smokers in a restaurant, but I know how it affects me!** (a former smoker)*

*****

It's not much fun to be a smoker in today's society. *Of course, I guess that something so harmful to one's health shouldn't be fun. (a smoker who can't quit)*

*****

I realize that I have most often been the silent victim because of innocence or ignorance about my reactions to smoking. *I am also disturbed by the violent expression of emotional energy that often accompanies my attempts to defend my own rights. Even as I try to confront people gently and non-threateningly, I probably radiate some sort of inner anger.* ***I still see smokers as a kind of lower caste, like the untouchables of India.*** *(a lifelong nonsmoker)*

*****

Nonsmokers have the right to be in a smoke-free environment, but only to a certain extent. Designated smoking areas are appropriate in restaurants, clubs and even office buildings. Smoke-free public buildings infringe on my rights. My taxes help pay for those buildings as well. *Private businesses have the right to be smoke-free, like McDonald's and Taco Bell, but I also have the privilege of not patronizing them. On one hand I feel like a lowdown, inferior person, but on the other hand I feel like someone unafraid to exert my rights. (a smoker who can't quit)*

*****

When my nonsmoking friends start in on smoking, I've been known to tell them, "Just wait, you're next." When they look mystified I say, "Well, you like your gin and tonic in the evening and insist on your wine with dinner. How do you know that the do-gooders aren't going to target you for consuming alcohol next?" *Responses have ranged from thoughtful to, "Well, at least my consuming alcohol doesn't hurt anyone else, like second-hand smoke." And I reply, "Ah, but health care and insurance costs are more for smokers. The next thing is alcohol-related diseases are on the rise and we're going to start charging you more." (a smoker who can't quit)*

*****

I will stop smoking when and if I decide to stop. I will not stop because someone else says I should, or because it's not politically correct. ***I consider this my individual right, and I choose to use tobacco.*** *(an unrepentant smoker)*

*****

I have lived with much unspoken resentment about smoking. People who don't want it around them are afraid to say anything—myself included. *Smokers who know they are offending others do it anyway, trying to ignore their comments and stares. Now I have guilt, remorse and frustration. One* *vivid memory illustrates this point: I'm holding my three-week-old, firstborn son in an elevator. A man lights up his cigarette and my son sneezes constantly for the duration of the ride. The smoker never seemed to notice the connection; he just kept puffing away. But I did not point-blank ask him to stop, which I should have. However, I did try to shield my son from the smoke and exited quickly, hoping the man would get the message. He didn't. (a former smoker)*

*****

I think raising taxes on tobacco is a politically popular idea. I do not believe that the additional taxes raised will be used to increase smoking cessation programs or to fund the additional medical costs that smokers incur. ***How popular would it be to raise taxes on fat- or sugar-laden products to discourage the use of those? Would those taxes be set aside to fund the additional medical costs incurred by excessive use of those items? I doubt it.*** *(a smoker who can't quit)*

*****

I would like all people to be extended the same courtesy l extend to nonsmokers: common courtesy, an acknowledgment that I might like to smoke, and a clue as to where it would be appropriate*, that is, "Oh, I have put an ashtray on the patio for you for whenever you would like to smoke." Wouldn't that be nice? (a smoker who can't quit)*

*****

There are things that smokers could have done, but I think it's too late now. ***Rude and messy smokers have made it tough on all of us:*** *People who toss burning cigarettes just anywhere, people who do not empty and clean ashtrays often enough in their houses and whose clothes get "that smell," people who light up while other people are still eating and people who smoke in cars with nonsmokers. (a smoker who can't quit)*

*****

I'm starting to feel like a social outcast. I feel like a fool standing out in the freezing cold smoking. *I'm smoking now as I write this. I've had eight cigarettes in the past hour since I came home from work. I'm angry that there are so many places you can't smoke and I'm furious when people are upset about my smoking. I think smokers are to be pitied. I'm angry because my husband thinks I can quit smoking because he did—my smoking is increasingly annoying him. Many of my friends have the same problem with their husbands. (a smoker who can't quit)*

*****

My own children say, in a nutshell, that people shouldn't smoke. I am proud of them since the ones who say this don't smoke themselves. One child and one in-law said that instead of smoking they enjoy wine for pleasure and to alleviate tension. ***I guess if I were perfect I wouldn't smoke and I wouldn't need a substitute. I know I am more comfortable risking the hazards of smoking than the hazards of alcohol or drugs.*** *Tobacco advertising is misleading, as are many other advertisements. I have never seen a tobacco ad show a person with emphysema. Nor have I ever seen an ad for alcohol show a person driving an automobile under the influence, much less a person with delirium tremens. I have never seen a high-fat food ad show a person suffering a heart attack or any other problem caused by atherosclerosis. I have never seen a high-sugar product ad show a person in diabetic shock or suffering amputation of the lower extremities because of diabetes. (a smoker who can't quit)*

*****

My best anti-tobacco experience, though, was riding a Greyhound bus. I was so mad I could have bit nails. I rode for twenty-seven hours. We had very few rest stops and we were running late so the stops were even shorter than usual. We broke down for three hours with no heat in seven-degree weather. I couldn't get off the bus and smoke, and I couldn't smoke on the bus. The guy sitting next to me was sitting happily chewing his tobacco and spitting wads on the floor of the bus. This was allowed because he wasn''t smoking. I guess the wads on the floor were not as disturbing to other passengers as second-hand smoke would be. When we got to the bus station, I was told I could not smoke inside the building. ***It's maddening—I paid the same price for my ticket as everyone else; however, their rights were considered more important than mine were. I did not recognize any of them as saints or royalty or anything. Why were they considered more important or better than I?*** *I now live in the tobacco belt of the United States so things are not so bad. (an unrepentant smoker)*

*****

A coworker once told me I needed a psychiatrist because I asked him, politely, to smoke elsewhere. (I had to be in the files that day, there were plenty of places for him to move to, and I offered to help him move his stuff.) I thought about what he said; I fully realize that part of my aversion to smoking stems from my perception of smoke and that it isn't totally due to my allergies. BUT WHY SHOULD I SEE A PSYCHIATRIST TO LEARN TO ACCEPT INHALING TOXINS AND CARCINOGENS? (a lifelong nonsmoker)

*****

I have written letters to the editor of my local newspaper, resulting in a storm of protest from the tobacco proponents, including invitations to get out of town and ply my trade in an area of more like-minded individuals, such as Boston. ***I may as well have attacked Mom, the Flag and Apple Pie.*** *Letters to my representatives usually go unanswered or result in a brief reproach. (a lifelong nonsmoker)*

*****

Many people today cry out that they have as much right to smoke as the nonsmoker to not smoke. I would concur, the smoker does have a right, but does it become a right for him to smoke and become party to mass genocide? *If smokers have the constitutional right to smoke and the courts allow them this right then the courts are condoning the annihilation of mankind. The constitution allows for citizens the right to bear arms, but this right is taken away from me because I'm a convicted felon. The same principle should be applied to the person who smokes: he smokes, thus*

*****

Most people who use tobacco today have jobs, support families, pay taxes, serve in the military, support the government and try to live the American dream. *It is hard for us to see the evil of smoking in today's society. Smoking doesn't even compare to abortion on demand, drug dealers walking the streets, murder, rape, robbery, crooked politicians, child murderers, HIV/AIDS, drunk drivers and so on. (an unrepentant smoker)*

*****

The tobacco user today has become a scapegoat for many people who see it as the cause of many of society's evils. *I don't condone tobacco use for everyone; it should be the individual's choice.* ***Some "experts" equate smokers and drug addicts. This may be politically correct, but it doesn't come from fact.*** *Smokers don't kill people or rob them to buy another smoke. Restrict smoking, sure. Consolidate it to certain areas, outlaw it in enclosed spaces and ban it in public places; however, when you treat smokers as criminals or lower-class humans you infringe on our individual rights and make us more resistant to change.* ***Some people react to smokers negatively, even though smoke doesn't bother them in any way. It is just socially correct in today's society to be negative to smokers.*** *(an unrepentant smoker)*

*****

In the early days when people began asking me not to smoke in their presence, the first few seemed hostile and aggressive—unnecessarily so. I have never been pleased to be the target of that sort of behavior. *I don't remember* *this happening in years, however, because I smoke in designated smoking areas or inquire if smoking bothers anyone in social situations without marked designated smoking areas, such as people's homes (including my own when I have guests). I don't smoke around people with medical conditions that would be aggravated by smoke, or around people who just don't like to be exposed to cigarette smoke. I would like those who don't like smoking to be as considerate of me as I am of them. Regulations restricting smoking in public places are fine with me, but in a few public buildings the designated smoking area is so poorly ventilated and the air there so unpleasant that I choose to go outdoors to smoke or postpone smoking altogether. Obviously, it does concentrate the unpleasantness of smoking to limit it to small, poorly ventilated areas that serve a large number of smokers. (a smoker who can't quit)*

*****

I don't smoke around guests who don't smoke. ***I respect nonsmokers. Too bad we don't get the same respect.*** *I have no problem not smoking in restaurants—if my guests do not smoke. I do, however, have a problem with holier-than-thou nonsmokers giving me advice on my private life. If anyone who feels this way visits my home, I tell them that if they do not want to smoke, they will have to not smoke outside. My eldest sister does not allow smoking in her house. Therefore, neither my parents nor I visit her, and she rarely visits us. (a smoker who can't quit)*

*****

You have to remember that smoking is legal. *I don't believe anyone should be trying to stop others from smoking in their presence. If the room is well ventilated there is no need to treat cigarette smokers as lepers. That's exactly the way we treat them. Now they have passed legislation so that the only public place they can smoke is outside. I feel bad for them. Quitting smoking is hard enough, but then you have to deal with people harassing you. It's not right. (a former smoker)*

*****

I have been exposed to secondhand smoke most of my life, at various jobs and in my own home. For the past several years I have forbidden smoke in my home. About eight years ago I became Prednisone dependent and shortly thereafter I had to retire from my last job. Now I avoid smokers whenever possible. When I had to endure other smokers the last few years before I had to quit work, I would ask them not to smoke around me. But I was the one who had to isolate myself. I had a woman blow smoke directly in my face at lunch one day; she's lucky I had enough self-control not to deck her. ***It has hurt and frustrated me—it has often brought me to tears.*** *(a former smoker)*

*****

Live and let live is what I say; *I am not my brother's keeper. I have tried to talk to alcoholics who were a danger to their families and innocent people by drinking and driving. We are all perfect children of God. I believe in abortion by choice, gay rights, the right to bear arms to protect one's family, interracial marriage, and smoker's rights. This country was founded on the principle that all persons were entitled to life, liberty, and the pursuit of happiness. And justice for all! Equally! (an unrepentant smoker)*

*****

Two years ago I lived next door to a woman who did not smoke. She did, however, use an oxygen mask when it suited her, and had her child skip school to do her shopping. Her child did all of her housework, laundry and cooking. Her only problem was that she was two hundred pounds overweight. All of her medical bills were paid by the welfare system. I could not smoke in the welfare office, but she could munch on chips and candy bars. And the government screams that my smoking is ruining my health! I haven't needed a doctor in six years I'll bet that if she has a heart attack it will be blamed on my secondhand smoke. Maybe the government should do a study on how obesity affects a person's health. ***Despite all of the dirty looks, nasty comments and the government trying to ban me from smoking in my own bathroom, until there are signs saying no fries or candy to overweight people in all public places, I will continue to be a happy smoker.*** *(an unrepentant smoker)*

*****

It is interesting to me that all tobacco use is apparently considered unacceptable to tobacco opponents. It is as if all tobacco use is tobacco abuse; a much different standard is applied to the use of alcohol or junk foods, for instance. *It is very difficult for most of us to control our use of tobacco, and those who can control their use probably set a frustrating example for those of us who can't, in the same way that occasional and moderate users of alcohol set a frustrating example for immoderate users. (a smoker who can't quit)*

*****

I am now seventy and have lived through all the scientific studies on meat, saccharine and alcohol, and I find that one by one they fall by the wayside. It seems to me that our country must have someone to hate; it makes people feel superior. First the Indians, then the Blacks, followed by Jews, Catholics, Mexicans, Asians and so on. ***The Civil Rights Movement made discrimination punishable by law, but aren't we smokers being discriminated against in a terrible way? Where are OUR rights to life, liberty and happiness?*** *(an unrepentant smoker)*

*****

Our president is now pushing a national health plan that will devastate the working classes—proposing a $1.00 per pack tax on cigarettes and a slight increase on alcohol taxes. Where are the surveys showing how many are killed each year in alcohol-related accidents versus so called "cigarette-induced cancers"? One by one our rights are being taken away by "Big Brother" mandating seat belts, motorcycle helmets, and a smoke-free nation. ***Alcohol should be taxed by volume at the same percentage proposed for cigarettes, but since alcohol consumption is an accepted social pastime comparable to tea drinking in England, and since our politicians have a high degree of alcoholism amongst them, equal taxation for tobacco and alcohol will not be considered appropriate.*** *May I add that while my husband and I do not drink beer or alcohol we do serve them in our home to our friends who indulge. We do not consider ourselves "better" because we do not drink. (an unrepentant smoker)*

*****

Stories

I Have Always Believed and Practiced Tolerance. I Am No One's Judge—A Smoker Who Believes She Can't Quit

I am constantly tormented about my smoking. In 1980, they found a tumor in my lung; fortunately, it calcified before the lung had to be removed. I did try to stop smoking: "cold turkey," acupuncture, patches. Nothing worked. Frankly, the withdrawal symptoms were a nightmare of the worst kind: My mind would not function; I felt as though I was in a tunnel and couldn't focus mentally on everyday tasks. It was agony, as well as frightening.

I once wondered what would happen if I had to choose between smoking and my husband of twenty years. His early death solved that problem. Between 1980 and 1984 when he died, I smoked outside; never when he was around. My husband was a health nut—he ran five miles a day and ate fish. He didn't smoke and died at forty-four.

I started smoking when I was old enough to find rabbit tobacco in the fields and started smoking regularly at sixteen when I went to a girl's boarding school. Both of my roommates smoked. I smoked in front of my parents and grandparents. It was a way of life for people who lived in North Carolina. They allowed smoking at school, but expelled anyone caught chewing gum instantly.

It was the thing to do. I bought cigarettes in every color to match my outfits. Can't you see me now? Sixteen years old, a size eight, straw hat, white gloves, suit, heels, hose and cigarettes to match: "Ain't she sweet?"

I encouraged both of my children to stay away from tobacco. I stressed this often and my son who is a dentist has never smoked. My daughter will smoke a cigarette or two each month if she is under stress. As an adult, that's her choice now, not mine.

Smoking is an individual's choice. I have always believed and practiced tolerance; I am no one's judge. We live in a free society. I resent legislation against tobacco products. I had much rather see a tobacco advertisement than a sex-related advertisement. I am tolerant and respect the rights of mankind.

I have several times cared for the dying and I didn't think about smoke, nicotine, lifestyles or anything else. It did not matter why they were dying—my focus was always on the person. I am not an "I told you so" person. I am tolerant of people and their habits or beliefs. I have been around cancer patients. Their physical agony was caused by the medical world. The ones I know who refused medical help died a quiet, dignified death. That's true of many terminal illnesses; otherwise, we would not have the Hemlock Society or Doctor Kevorkian. Grief is grief. It's ridiculous to lump grief and tobacco together; so many people want to blame something.

Today I have a different problem. My son-in-law is completely intolerant of everything, including my smoking, unless he wants to leave the children at my house. Fortunately, he lives in the same town now, but next year the family moves to Texas. I will never stay in my daughter's home because of her husband's feelings about smoking. I am stubborn, but I'm also angry. Two of my best friends who also smoke have been hospitalized for long-term care. Both have been denied patches or any help to combat their nicotine dependency and both have deteriorated mentally. Both were medicated with Prozac. That is not the answer, but the medical world does not care about smokers.

Why don't I stop smoking? I am not willing to go through that agony again. Besides, as I said, I am stubborn. I like my life and my lifestyle. My doctor bills run about $300 a year. Last year it was ear infections and a blocked tear duct. Frankly, I can live in my own world without sanctimonious do-gooders who spend time traveling in exhaust fumes, barbecuing fillets and complaining about secondhand smoke. Does the rise in cost hurt me? Not really, I'll just contribute less to the church and buy more cigarettes. Am I a cynic? I think not, but I am a problem that represents the lifestyles of the past.

I Have Never Seen a Tobacco Ad Show a Person with Emphysema—A Smoker Who Won't Quit

It really is vastly different to be a tobacco user in today's society as compared to that of the early 1960s when tobacco use was almost universally tolerated and generally condoned.

Increased education about the hazards of tobacco use is important today, and I appreciate the fact that many young people have, by means of this education, decided not to take up smoking. My husband and I have a combined family of seven grown children; of the seven, only three have tried smoking, and only one remains a smoker at this time.

As a tobacco user in today's society, I am glad that there is more information available about the effects of its use and glad that there is greater protection for nonsmokers. I would like to see greater protection from alcohol and other substance abuse as well, and I am very distressed that our very own government promotes the use of condoms as "safe" sex, disregarding the physical and spiritual hazards of such a claim.

Both my parents smoked and thought it was all right for grownups to smoke. They emphasized that I should not smoke until I graduated from high school for health reasons. I might have smoked four cigarettes in high school when friends offered them to me, but I was not really interested in smoking then. I began to smoke soon after high school graduation—I had earned the right. It seemed that most adults smoked then.

My parents did not make me smoke, but after I took it up my father gave me two lovely cigarette lighters and my mother gave me a lovely silver cigarette case. I don't remember there being any trouble between smokers and nonsmokers in those days.

My father had moderate emphysema. He died of a heart attack, but had quit smoking twelve years before. His family had a history of death by heart attacks. He was seventy and lived longer than other of his family members, none of whom smoked to my knowledge. My mother and two brothers died at sixty-five of heart problems that I believe were tobacco-related among other causative factors.

There was nothing to encourage me not to smoke. It is now pretty solidly built into my lifestyle, and I consider it my bad habit of choice. It wasn't until the mid-1960s that my doctor said more or less that smoking is bad for health, and that I shouldn't do it. But when he checked my heart and lungs they were in excellent condition, and nothing more was said. He and other doctors then considered a pack a day reasonable. By then I had discovered on my own that excessive smoking is unhealthy and, therefore, unpleasant. I worked out my own ways to limit smoking to a level that I considered acceptable for the most part. I quit for ten weeks and gained fifteen pounds—and I missed smoking. Later I had successfully reduced my smoking to five cigarettes a day and sustained that level for weeks. But then I suddenly faced an unavoidable and serious crisis and found that increased smoking calmed me. I have been able to reduce my consumption to five a day three or four times since then. The last time was a year ago—again, I started to increase my consumption after an unavoidable and serious crisis. The doggone things are calming, and I enjoy a few of them regularly when things are calm as well. I'm making progress now, reducing again from ten to fifteen a day and hoping eventually to get back to five a day.

In the early days when people began asking me not to smoke in their presence, the first few seemed hostile and aggressive—unnecessarily so. I have never been pleased to be the target of that sort of behavior. I don't remember this happening in years, however, because I smoke in designated smoking areas or inquire if smoking bothers anyone in social situations without marked designated smoking areas, such as people's homes (including my own when I have guests). I don't smoke around people with medical conditions that would be aggravated by smoke, or around people who just don't like to be exposed to cigarette smoke. I would like those who don't like smoking to be as considerate of me as I am of them.

Regulations restricting smoking in public places are fine with me, but in a few public buildings the designated smoking area is so poorly ventilated and the air there so unpleasant that I choose to go outdoors to smoke or postpone smoking altogether. Obviously, it does concentrate the unpleasantness of smoking to limit it to small, poorly ventilated areas that serve a large number of smokers.

I think raising taxes on tobacco is a politically popular idea. I do not believe that the additional taxes raised will be used to increase smoking cessation programs or to fund the additional medical costs that smokers incur. How popular would it be to raise taxes on fat- or sugar-laden products to discourage the use of those? Would those taxes be set aside to fund the additional medical costs incurred by excessive use of those items? I doubt it.

My own children say, in a nutshell, that people shouldn't smoke. I am proud of them since the ones who say this don't smoke themselves. One child and one in-law said that instead of smoking they enjoy wine for pleasure and to alleviate tension. I guess if I were perfect I wouldn't smoke and I wouldn't need a substitute. I know I am more comfortable risking the hazards of smoking than the hazards of alcohol or drugs.

Tobacco advertising is misleading, as are many other advertisements. I have never seen a tobacco ad show a person with emphysema. Nor have I ever seen an ad for alcohol that shows a person driving an automobile under the influence, much less a person with delirium tremens. I have never seen a high-fat food ad show a person suffering a heart attack or any other problem caused by atherosclerosis. I have never seen a high-sugar product ad show a person in diabetic shock or suffering amputation of the lower extremities because of diabetes.

I agree with restrictions to protect young people from tobacco use. A young person can develop better without tobacco. Also, if a person reaches full maturity without the use of tobacco as well as other habituating or addictive substances, he or she may well have developed sufficient coping mechanisms to manage without them permanently. Of course, there is still the danger of tobacco and alcohol becoming part of rites of passage into adulthood.

Smoking is pleasurable. I have used it as a reward for completing a certain number of tasks or when sitting and thinking or listening…

I Will Try in the Future to Think of Smokers as Victims Rather Than Aggressors—A Lifelong Nonsmoker

It never occurred to me that everyone's eyes did not burn most of the time. I was totally unaware of how tobacco smoke was affecting my life until the damage was done. I am not and never have been a smoker, but I did live my first thirty-five years with smokers at home, at school, and at work. As a child, I had many respiratory ailments, including pneumonia at eighteen.

There is a family story about attempts to take me for car rides when I was an infant. I would always get sick and throw up on someone. Only in retrospect has it become clear to me that the reason I was sick was that one or more people in the car would have been smoking. I still get nauseated when in a car with smokers, but at least now I am able to make my needs known.

My father was a pipe and cigar smoker. On a vacation trip by car in my mid-twenties, I felt nauseated every day after lunch. On the second day, I realized my reaction was related to father's smoking. He stopped smoking in the car, and I did not have the problem again.

Since reaching thirty-five, I've organized my life to omit smokers. This means that my social contacts are mainly limited to nonsmokers. I avoid all social gatherings where smoking is allowed. The effects of other people's smoke have always clouded my enjoyment of movies and other public events. Now, in California and other places, smoke-free public places have greatly helped me enjoy life. There still remains the fact that even if one chooses to eat at an outdoor facility, smokers may still be upwind of your space and therefore render your meal only marginally enjoyable.

At one time I lived in downtown San Francisco and walked to work, about eight blocks away. Very often I would see burned mattresses in the street—silent evidence of a smoker's night dance with death, endangering not just their own lives but the lives of many others in the neighborhood.

Right now, I live in a senior community of single-floor dwellings, and fortunately, the closest smoker is across the street. Still, I can occasionally smell the smoke of his cigarette; he is outside a lot of the time. Almost every place I have ever lived has been invaded by a neighbor's smoke. In apartments, it creeps up in the plumbing spaces and often goes out one person's window and into another person's. Does it always have to be mine?

Another lifelong occurrence is going to restaurants to eat and then coming home to find that you have brought home the smoke-filled stench of the restaurant. Even your hair seems to absorb the smoke smell within a fairly short time.

Most public places provide ample opportunity for conflicts with smokers, and those in authority are often too timid or lacking in motivation to keep a space smoke-free. I can't blame them; challenging a person's right to smoke is always like setting off an emotional firebomb.

I realize that I have most often been the silent victim because of innocence or ignorance about my reactions to smoking. I am also disturbed by the violent expression of emotional energy that often accompanies my attempts to defend my own rights. Even as I try to confront people gently and nonthreateningly, I probably radiate some sort of inner anger. I still see smokers as a kind of lower caste, like the untouchables of India.

Thinking about my life, I realize that my worst moments connected with smoke occurred when I was hospitalized with a ruptured appendix. While I was being transported from one floor to another (barely alive with peritonitis) via the elevator, many people got on including a doctor—carrying a lit cigarette! I was too ill to complain, but I did get a good look at him. Several months later while returning to the hospital for tests, I got on the elevator and he was the only one other person on it with me. I took advantage of the situation to lecture him on the need to observe the safety laws prohibiting smoking in elevators as well as the laws of human kindness regarding patients who might be desperately ill.

Immediately after my operation (maybe five days), they were taking a new patient's information, with the intent of putting her in the same room with me. When I heard that she smoked one-and-a-half packs a day I rose out of my sickbed and went to the nurses' station demanding that they get "that woman" out of my room. All in all, hospitals were then rotten places to try to get well.

I tried to encourage several friends or associates to quit smoking; I was struck by how hesitant they were to the idea. Now I realize that they were so addicted that it was a real hardship for them to consider giving it up. Having never smoked, I did not realize the problem they faced.

I Got a Lot More Work Done When I Could Smoke at My Desk—A Smoker Who Can't Quit

The only way smoking has affected my life is the controversy over it. I was very upset when my job started a no-smoking policy. What bothered me the most was people at work saying how glad they were that people could not smoke in their office anymore when no one smoked in their office in the first place. I got a lot more work done when I could smoke at my desk. After the policy was enforced, I took my breaks.

It bothers me when alcoholics or people who drink and drive tell me not to smoke because of the harm I am doing to myself. It bothers me when obese people give me the same advice. The people that I know who died of cancer never smoked a day in their life.

I don't smoke around guests who don't smoke. I respect nonsmokers. Too bad we don't get the same respect.

I have no problem not smoking in restaurants if my guests do not smoke. I do, however, have a problem with holier-than-thou nonsmokers giving me advice on my private life. If anyone who feels this way visits my home, I tell them that if they do not want to smoke, they will have to not smoke outside. My eldest sister does not allow smoking in her house. Therefore, neither my parents nor I visit her, and she rarely visits us.

I quit smoking for six months after I had back surgery and then picked up the habit again after gaining too much weight. I worked out for five days a week and could not lose the weight.

I realize that I am addicted. Each time I quit I start up again, and the craving is always there.

My Doctor Suggested That I Take Up Smoking—An Unrepentant Smoker

I didn't start smoking until after my children were born. I don't think it would have damaged them had I done so. I think our bodies adjust to whatever environment we grow up in. If they didn't, our species would have died out long ago.

When I was twenty-nine years old—widowed with three sons, ages four, seven and eight—I became extremely nervous and compulsive. My doctor prescribed a tranquilizer, but after using them for a few weeks I refused to take them since they left me groggy and unable to care for my children adequately. My doctor asked me if I smoked and suggested that I take up smoking. When I felt myself becoming stressed, he said, just sit down, smoke a cigarette and relax. It worked! And it was an acceptable social practice; everyone smoked in the fifties, and I have smoked every day (1 1/2 packs of cigarettes a day) since then.

Thirty-five years ago, I had a hysterectomy for cancer of the cervix and now I am fine, very active and healthy—thank God!

My entire life has been devoted to children. I raised my children alone for fourteen years and chose not to marry again until they had all left home. My two oldest sons have master's degrees and my youngest son went into the military. I have now been married for twenty-six years to my second husband, who also loves children. In the past twenty-five years, we have helped to raise five children from broken homes—they are all now healthy and successful. (We are not foster parents; the state does not compensate us for our expenditures.)

We now have an eight-year-old boy from an unmarried mother who came to us when he was eight weeks old so that his mother could complete her high school education. She is on welfare and has had a second child by a different father but is still unmarried. We do not ask compensation for his care.

None of my sons smoke. The eight-year-old and I have a pact: I will not smoke while he's sitting on my lap or in his bedroom as long as he does his homework with a smile. Whenever he starts to object to homework I just pick up my cigarette package and he says, "No! No! I'll do it, and I'll smile."

I am now seventy plus and have lived through all the scientific studies on meat, saccharine and alcohol, and I find that one by one they fall by the wayside. It seems to me that our country must have someone to hate; it makes people feel superior. First the Indians, then the Blacks, followed by Jews, Catholics, Mexicans, Asians and so on. The Civil Rights Movement made discrimination punishable by law, but aren't we smokers being discriminated against in a terrible way? Where are our rights to life, liberty and happiness?

Our president is now pushing a national health plan that will devastate the working classes—proposing a significant per pack tax on cigarettes and a slight increase in alcohol taxes. Where are the surveys showing how many are killed each year in alcohol-related accidents versus so-called cigarette-induced cancers? One by one our rights are being taken away by "Big Brother" mandating seat belts, motorcycle helmets, and a smoke-free nation.

Alcohol should be taxed by volume at the same percentage proposed for cigarettes, but since alcohol consumption is an accepted social pastime comparable to tea drinking in England, and since our politicians have a high degree of alcoholism among them, equal taxation for tobacco and alcohol will not be considered appropriate. May I add that while my husband and I do not drink beer or alcohol we do serve them in our home to our friends who indulge. We do not consider ourselves "better" because we do not drink.

How have cigarettes affected our lives? We have a son who lives in Atlanta, Georgia, whom we love very much. He has a lovely wife and a six-year-old son, whom we truly love. We used to visit with them every Christmas and I flew back every summer to spend time with our grandchild while they went on vacation. My daughter-in-law forbids smoking in her home and I respect her wishes; however, December in Atlanta is not the best time to be smoking outdoors. Once, while sitting in their snow-filled patio having a cigarette and nursing a terrible cold, I decided that I would not visit them again and I haven't, giving one excuse after another for our absences.

Every summer they fly the little boy to us. We have him for three weeks while they go on vacation. We love it. We take him and our eight-year-old on vacation. This year we left August 30th and returned home September 14th. We went to San Diego, to the zoo, Sea World, Wild Animal Park, on to La Jolla to the aquarium and to the Los Angeles area where we picked up a second grandchild and went to Universal Studios, Knott's Berry Farm and Magic Mountain. All in two weeks time—not bad for a seventy-year-old grandmother who smokes! And I enjoyed every moment of the hectic trip. Isn't it ironic that while I may not smoke in my son's home, they willingly send their only child into our smoke-filled home for three weeks at a time?

I do not encourage smoking. I tell everyone it's a nasty, dirty habit—your hair smells and your clothes smell and your breath is terrible. It's a bad habit and I love it.

Living in Nevada where smoking is permissible in casinos, I am often berated by other gamblers for smoking. Not long ago a lady objected to my smoking so I extinguished my cigarette; yet she went on and on about how cigarette smoke would kill me and that I had no right to subject her to secondhand smoke and endanger her health, that "those cigarettes" would hasten her death. I was embarrassed beyond words by her loud vocal abuse. When I could stand it no longer I said to her, "Madam, I was smoking when you sat down next to me, so you made your choice. I'm sorry that my smoking offends you, but if I were as worried about my health as you seem to be, and if I were truly worried about death as you seem to be, and if I were you, I'd go home and lose thirty pounds." Needless to say, she left.

The secret to a long and happy life is to remove stress, help others, relax and trust in God. A sense of humor is an added asset. I'm certain you will receive many letters filled with heartaches and pathos, all due to the evils of tobacco. Here's a happy letter from a little old lady in tennis shoes who refuses to get old and turns her back on the paranoia that grips our nation. During my last medical check-up my doctor said, "Marne, you're amazing. You'll live another sixteen years." Well, that's all I ask. Our eight-year-old should be done with college by that time.

Live and let live is what I say; I am not my brother's keeper. I have tried to talk to alcoholics who were a danger to their families and innocent people by drinking and driving. We are all perfect children of God. I believe in abortion by choice, gay rights, the right to bear arms to protect one's family, interracial marriage and smoker's rights. This country was founded on the principle that all persons were entitled to life, liberty, and the pursuit of happiness. And justice for all! Equally!

"Call Dr. X. I Don't Treat Patients Who Smoke!"—A Former Smoker

I'm fifty-three years old. I smoked for about thirty years until I had my first heart attack in January 1988. If I had known the actual consequences of smoking, I would have quit years ago. Unfortunately, I ignored those who kept encouraging me to quit.

I'm now in prison, serving eleven years for theft and forgery and, unfortunately, I'm being subjected to secondhand smoke. I've had doctor's orders to be placed in a nonsmoking unit, but the prison doesn't have one. I'm suffering from all the smoke in the air because of my coronary and artery disease. I have filed a 1983 Civil Rights Act Complaint raising the issue of environmental tobacco smoke (E.T.S.), but it will be years before it comes to trial. By that time I'll be released, or possibly dead. I've written to the governor, to newspapers, the Department of Corrections and other agencies, but none have responded.

I'm now in the process of filing a lawsuit against the eight major tobacco companies for producing and selling tobacco products. I've got the paperwork prepared, but I cannot find an attorney to handle it for me on a contingency basis. I can't afford to hire an attorney as I make only thirteen dollars a month for my prison labor, and out or that meager stipend I need to purchase my medications, toiletry items, commissary, postage and other incidentals.

To make matters worse, besides having to breathe secondhand smoke, I have to live among people with tuberculosis, hepatitis, AIDS, herpes, and other unchecked communicable diseases.

To be a tobacco smoker in today's society shows a complete disregard and disrespect for one's health. I was a two- to three-pack-a-day smoker for over thirty years and did not heed the advice of anyone about the dangers of smoking. I smoked Camels and always enjoyed their tobacco; I didn't realize they added hundreds of other chemicals to their tobacco. I acted immaturely when people attempted to educate me about the potential hazards of smoking, not only to my own health but also to those around me exposed to my secondhand smoke.

Over the years I became addicted to cigarettes, thinking they were enjoyable. As I got older I watched relatives and friends succumb to lung cancer and it set off an alarm in my brain. Attempting several times to quit smoking I found that I actually craved cigarettes and nicotine. My body would scream out at me, "Hey! You better not deprive me of nicotine!"

After my second heart attack, I lay in the hospital emergency room, hooked up to a plethora of machines. The doctor attending to my needs looked at my shirt pocket and saw my cigarettes. "You smoke?" he inquired. When I replied in the affirmative he looked at a nurse and said "Call Doctor X. I don't treat patients who smoke!" Then he left the emergency room. I quit again, but within six months I was back to my two- to three-pack-a-day habit. I was weak, tired, and could not hold down a job. I had to ask for welfare, which gave me food stamps but no other assistance. Social Security denied me any help—I was told to change my occupation.

So I did, to that of an artist—check artist, that is! And, well, you know the rest of the story. After imprisonment and suffering yet another heart attack, I made up my mind to quit. I opened my cans of tobacco and dumped them down my commode, which blew my cellmate's mind. He smoked more than I did.

Trying to quit when everyone else around you smokes and you have no place to go is hard. In prison, it was really tough. The withdrawals were painful. I was edgy and nervous. I was addicted. Even when I was almost out of money, I would spend it on cigarettes instead of food. When I quit

I actually developed an eating disorder; I ate to replace smoking. I ended up with a thirty-six-inch waist—picked up about thirty pounds. I quit in June of 1991. I haven't had two cigarettes since. Now, after going on a crusade to ban smoking in the prison, I have become somewhat of a dirty taste in other people's mouths. After I quit I filed an injunction in Federal Court ordering the prison to place me in a nonsmoking area. The prison does not have a nonsmoking area, and I'm now in Federal Court suing the Department of Corrections to open a nonsmoking unit. The prison staff has labeled me a "nit-picker" and a "troublemaker."

Not having the money to hire an attorney I had to proceed pro se. It's like David and Goliath. I can't even use the law library now because they moved me to a medical unit, and we aren't allowed to go anywhere. They did this to prevent me from properly attacking the smoking issue. They will probably have the court dismiss my lawsuit.

If I knew about the actual impurities in tobacco twenty years ago I would have quit then! I didn't know that more than 4000 chemical compounds have been identified in tobacco smoke, at least forty-three of which are known to cause cancer in humans. Plus, each year secondhand smoke kills over 3000 adult nonsmokers from lung cancer.

Today's smokers are more educated than those twenty to thirty years ago, and knowing all the hazards of smoking, the smoker today should be eager to quit. Smoking has lessened somewhat in America, but the tobacco moguls are now concentrating on foreign markets where smoking and the number of smokers have greatly increased.

A lot of taxes are derived from the sales of tobacco products, but that's a mere pittance compared to what it costs the taxpayers for the medical complications brought on by the use of tobacco products. I believe the politicians don't really care about the effects of tobacco smoking; they just want to raise taxes so they can continue to operate a corrupt government. I trust my fellow convicts more than I would most politicians.

Many people today cry out that they have as much right to smoke as the nonsmoker does to not smoke. I would concur; the smoker does have a right, but is it a right for him to become party to mass genocide? If smokers have the constitutional right to smoke and the courts allow them this right then the courts are condoning the annihilation of mankind. The constitution allows for citizens the right to bear arms, but this right is taken away from me because I'm a convicted felon. The same principle should be applied to the person who smokes: he smokes, thus contributing to killing innocent, passive inhalers, therefore his right should be taken from him.

In a nutshell, the government is concerned about baseball strikes, inhumane conditions and genocide in many foreign countries, yet it fails to take a positive stance on eliminating tobacco products.

After thirty years of smoking, I would encourage all smokers to quit! The tobacco companies should be compelled to pay for centers for the smokers to be treated for their tobacco addiction. The tobacco company titans should pay all the medical bills of any smoking-related illness.

It's Almost Like Ecstasy When I Light Up—An Unrepentant Smoker

I am a happy tobacco user. I have smoked for fifteen years. I thoroughly enjoy it and don't want to quit. I know all of the risks involved. I see them in my family every day. Many of my family have died from cancer. My father was a smoker and died recently from congestive heart failure, and my mother was a smoker and is now having radiation for lung cancer. I knew all of the risks before I started. I started smoking by lighting cigarettes for my mother and sneaking puffs. I was a regular smoker at seventeen.

I know the risks. I was a science and biology major in high school and college; I am not an ignorant person. In my hectic life, I enjoy taking a break and smoking a cigarette. I have two small children, and often a cigarette break is my only relaxation during the day.

It seems that over the last five years I have fewer and fewer rights. Nonsmokers are constantly complaining about secondhand smoke. I wonder if they have ever been in the same room with smokers who have not been able to smoke for a few hours. Which would be more detrimental to their health, the deprived smokers or the secondhand smoke?

I am angry that smokers are blamed for anything and everything—an unexplained fire? Obviously a careless smoker. You catch a cold? You have been around too much secondhand smoke. Never mind that it's flu season and you've kissed everyone in a one-mile radius. If you have a stressful day, you smoke too much.

I have sat in restaurants and gotten looks and comments that would kill because I lit a cigarette after dinner. I don't comment to anyone if they choose not to smoke. I feel I am looked at like I care nothing for my home, my family, my health or my children. I am treated like a contagious leper. The fact is that my home and family are my top priority. They are my life.

Many years ago in Salt Lake City, Utah, I was asked to leave a public restaurant for lighting a cigarette. I was so mad. My money is just as good as anyone else's! Yet I had to leave because I lit a cigarette.

I was having some coffee once at an outside cafe when my oldest child was a toddler. She reached for my lighter and I scolded her. A woman at the next table told me if I didn't have to smoke my child wouldn't accidentally burn herself playing with my lighter. I suppose I should also get rid of my kitchen stove so she couldn't burn herself on that either. I told the woman that, and the indignant look on her face was hilarious—I felt very justified in saying it and meant for her to know it.

My husband and I are both tobacco users and we lead a very active and physical life. We are much healthier than most people our age. Nonsmokers would have you believe all smokers are curled up in a fetal position with an oxygen mask from the age of twenty-five.

I've also noticed in public places that a man lighting a cigar or pipe doesn't get near the negativity as anyone lighting a cigarette. I don't know if it's usually men who have cigars or pipes and women don't, or if nonsmokers actually believe cigarettes are worse.

I was a bartender for about four years and I enjoyed it. I also noticed patterns in people's behaviors. If a stranger came in and they were just drinking they were pretty well left alone. If they were smoking, no matter what—a pipe, cigar, cigarettes—a conversation usually started. Maybe it was just a person asking for a light, but it was a conversation. A friend and I tried it as an experiment and it's true seventy-five percent of the time.

The workplace rules about smoking are a joke. Anymore you cannot smoke in any government building. I find it very strange that Mr. Clinton wanted to raise cigarette taxes to pay for health care reform, and yet also sought to ban smoking in all public places. It's like cutting off your nose to spite your face. Does the government honestly believe they can stop everyone from smoking or chewing tobacco?

At the last restaurant I worked in I could not smoke inside the building during working hours. I also did not get a break to go outside and smoke. The manager said it would be a bad influence on the teenagers I worked with. However, most of the teenagers lit up if the boss wasn't around. It was the biggest joke!

My best anti-tobacco experience, though, was riding a Greyhound bus. I was so mad I could have spit nails. I rode for twenty-seven hours. We had very few rest stops and we were running late so the stops were even shorter than usual. We broke down for three hours with no heat in seven-degree weather. I couldn't get off the bus and smoke, and I couldn't smoke on the bus. The guy sitting next to me was sitting happily chewing his tobacco and spitting wads on the floor of the bus. This was allowed because he wasn't smoking. I guess the wads on the floor were not as disturbing to other passengers as secondhand smoke would be. When we got to the bus station, I was told I could not smoke inside the building. It's maddening—I paid the same price for my ticket as everyone else; however, their rights were considered more important than mine were. I did not recognize any of them as saints or royalty or anything. Why were they considered more important or better than I? I now live in the tobacco belt of the USA so things are not so bad.

Two years ago I lived next door to a woman who did not smoke. However, she did use an oxygen mask when it suited her, and had her child skip school to do her shopping. Her child did all of her housework, laundry and cooking. Her only problem was that she was two hundred pounds overweight. All of her medical bills were paid by the welfare system. I could not smoke in the welfare office, but she could munch on chips and candy bars. And the government screams that my smoking is ruining my health! I haven't needed a doctor in six years. I'll bet that if she has a heart attack it will be blamed on my secondhand smoke. Maybe the government should do a study on how obesity affects a person's health.

Despite all of the dirty looks, nasty comments and the government trying to ban me from smoking in my own bathroom, until there are signs saying no fries or candy to overweight people in all public places, I will continue to be a happy smoker.

Yes, I am addicted. I like it very much and I don't want to quit. It's like ecstasy when I light up. If it is addiction, I am thoroughly enjoying it. At least my tobacco is legal.

CHAPTER 6

Health

Many smokers, especially those who don't want to quit, feel like they are the healthiest people they know; they justify their self-diagnoses, attributing any health problems, if they exist, to age. Frequently assertions include: "My children are healthy, and I smoked throughout my pregnancy" or, "I have never had a sick day in my life!" These statements are often accompanied by accounts of unhealthy nonsmokers, particularly the obese, whose habits smokers see as posing a comparable if not worse danger to one's health. Many smokers, whether or not they are trying to quit their habit are skeptical of scientific information, and information disseminated by the government. Words like "hysteria" and "paranoia" abound in the narratives of smokers, one even claiming that "if a person believes a practice to be harmful to him then that possibility exists."

It is impossible for smokers who deny the effects of tobacco use on their own health to acknowledge the effects of secondhand smoke to nonsmokers. Many dismiss the very real problems of allergies, respiratory ailments and so on that nonsmokers face when exposed to secondhand smoke, believing either that nonsmokers only hate smoke because they are allowed this right as a privileged majority, that these problems are exaggerated, or mere illusions.

Some smokers are very aware of the effects of secondhand smoke and feel guilty about their addictions, but helpless when confronted with the difficulties of quitting. Because many smokers come from smoking families, some of them acknowledge suffering from allergies and other respiratory ailments themselves due to secondhand smoke exposure as

I. Newman and J. DeFrain, *Tobacco Use and Intimate Relationships*,
https://doi.org/10.1007/978-3-319-92579-0_6

children and smoking as adults. For these smokers who do believe that smoking affects their health and the health of those around them, quitting is still a challenge, and fear for their health and the health of loved ones must compete with fear of going without tobacco. Unfortunately, because of the tenacity of addiction, many of these smokers do not quit until their worst fears are realized and they are confronted with a diagnosis of cancer or another smoke-related disease. For those that do quit, a few resume smoking because of weight gain, a fate apparently worse than smoke-related disease and death. The equation of weight and beauty as well as health in our society obviously has serious consequences to smokers and nonsmokers alike; one nonsmoker recalled that her doctor recommended she take up smoking to lose weight.

Nonsmokers and former smokers who suffer from allergies due to exposure to secondhand smoke describe in detail the history of their problems with tobacco, leaving no room for doubt that secondhand smoke constitutes a constant and imminent risk to their lives in myriad ways. Many have been subjected to secondhand smoke from childhood and recall the oppressive atmospheres they grew up in as directly responsible for chronic health problems that began when they were children. Several nonsmokers relate moving accounts of dealing with constant exposure to smoke in the workplace leading to chronic and worsening respiratory problems and even disability amid the disbelief and discrimination of smoking colleagues.

Smokers and nonsmokers alike generally feel that the medical establishment treats the issue of tobacco use ineffectively, inappropriately, and inhumanely. Smokers feel that doctors, nurses, and medical facilities fail to take into account the needs of smokers as addicts; many feel that such treatment is pure discrimination. Smokers and nonsmokers express the need for medical institutions to treat patients who smoke as people with addictions, rather than weak-willed, weak-minded tobacco abusers. Unfortunately, many smokers write of avoiding health checkups and care, because of constant questioning, denial of care and other "abuse" from doctors and nurses, a fact that may delay the decision to quit and the early detection and timely treatment of disease. For others, the insecurities and fears that come with dealing with addiction are exacerbated by what they see as constant harassment from physicians who attribute all their ailments to tobacco use and consistently advise patients to quit.

Nonsmokers, on the other hand, generally wish that physicians were more consistent about smoking, several complaining that physicians who cared for their smoking parent or family member did not take a stance against smoking and advise quitting. Smokers also complain of the excessive costs of programs to quit, counseling, aids, and other methods, none of which make their battle with addiction any easier. Nonsmokers also need recourse to affordable means of support, such as counseling and group therapy when dealing with a loved one's addiction, or the illness or death of a loved one.

Testimony

Some people react to smokers negatively, even though it doesn't bother them in any way. ***It is just socially correct in today's society to be negative to smokers.*** *(an unrepentant smoker)*

*****

Earlier I saw doctors for my addiction problems. I seriously considered counseling, but my medical program covers only 50 percent of ten sessions. Each session is $120 with an initial session of $150. ***I cannot afford to pay for the balance, and our medical insurance does not cover nicotine dependence counseling, patches, gum or any other wellness kind of program.*** *(a smoker who can't quit)*

*****

At twenty-nine I was finally diagnosed with asthma. Smoke is a particular irritant for me, even in the lightest concentrations. I have spent over ten years on medication, at times steroids, to be able to breathe. My asthma is very much under control now, but I can go nowhere without a nebulizer for fear smoke will shut down my lungs. (a lifelong nonsmoker)

*****

The doctors say that smoking did cause my husband's problems as well as my own! IS anybody listening? (a former smoker)

*****

Because tobacco smoke is everywhere I go, I cannot enjoy the many events I'd like to enjoy in my golden years. I cannot even spend a night at the home of my daughter or son because both my son and son-in-law smoke. I cannot breathe too well after visiting there during the day and have to go outside frequently. When they visit my home, they go outside to smoke. My two young grandchildren want us to spend Christmas Eve and Christmas Day with them. In order to do this I have to have cough syrup with codeine, which is difficult to get. My internist and my allergy specialist will not prescribe it because they are afraid of addiction. Also, due to the drug abuse in our society, the narcotic records of doctors and pharmacists are examined regularly. Whenever I ask at the pharmacy to sign for a preparation with codeine I'm very uncomfortable doing so and I don't like the treatment I get when I'm out of my home territory. They simply say, "I don't have any!" (a lifelong nonsmoker)

*****

I am certain that, although I have been "cured" of cancer, my life expectancy has been significantly reduced. *The normal life expectancy for healthy, white males is currently seventy-two years and here I am sixty-one already and realistically, not "healthy."* ***Tobacco use has exacted a big toll from my life and no doubt shortened what remains of it.*** *(a former smoker)*

*****

I quit smoking shortly after I retired and went from one hundred and thirty pounds on a five-foot, one-and-a-half inch frame to one hundred and seventy-eight pounds. I was miserable; I hated the fat, hated the way I looked and was a physically handicapped, depressed and unhappy person. So I started smoking again a year later. I am now one hundred and forty pounds and trying to keep the weight off. I walk at least a mile every day, move the twenty-, thirty- and forty-foot sprinklers on five and a half acres of pasture and garden and keep the house in good shape, all two thousand and five square feet of it. I find there is something to do from six in the morning till six at night, so I don't have time to watch news on TV or read the newspaper. You might say I wear out the knees of my pants more than I do the rear end because I am so active. (a smoker who can't quit)

*****

The hardest part of watching someone who is sick or dying from tobacco use is knowing that the illness and progression to death were preventable, that the horror of tobacco-induced illness and death was self-inflicted, caused by a loved one who smoked or was an occupational hazard of being chronically exposed to environmental tobacco smoke at work. (a lifelong nonsmoker)

*****

My first husband died of lung cancer at thirty-five. He was predisposed to cancer; his father died of cancer and his mother was treated for cancer. His brother died at twelve. He also worked in radar while in the military. I think genetics plays a large part in our health. *My present husband smokes. My best friend has never smoked and she would like me to quit for the sake of* *my health.* ***It is ironic that she has never smoked and has one health problem after another. I don't have any health problems.*** *(an unrepentant smoker)*

*****

My respiratory symptoms increased after two or three years in this very smoky atmosphere. When I could no longer sleep at night and my symptoms had become fairly chronic, I went to an allergist who diagnosed asthma and chronic severe rhinitis, sinusitis and pharyngitis. After taking my medical history and doing allergy tests, the doctor had no doubt that I was having a reaction to smoke. He offered to write a letter to my employer saying I needed to work in a nonsmoking environment, but I was embarrassed about it; I felt that smoke was just something I would have to tolerate as long as I worked. (a lifelong nonsmoker)

*****

I have enjoyed smoking for many years and have never considered it to be an addiction. This may not be true for other smokers. ***I believe that if a person believes a practice to be harmful to him then that possibility exists. With the hammering that the public gets from all sides on all matters of health, it is a great battle to stay healthy. I am healthy now. Any difficulties that I have are from the battering of my frame, which is still up and going. I think that it is extreme to say that so many diseases are caused by the use of tobacco. To me, a tobacco-caused illness is an uncertainty.*** *To me, smoking is not an addiction. Since we are all psychologically different I realize that to some people the use of tobacco may be an addiction. I am opposed to the U.S. government's use of power more than persuasion to deal with cigarettes. (an unrepentant smoker)*

*****

This [cancer] has devastated our lives. ***If only we had known what terrible destruction smoking could cause.*** *(a former smoker)*

*****

I started smoking at sixteen and am still enjoying it at seventy-four. I started by imitating my friends. ***I have never missed a day of work, rarely have colds and have only been in the hospital twice: forty years ago for a hernia and twenty-five years ago for pancreatitis. I am a fairly active person, taking care of my own lawn work, painting, car washing,* etc. *I play golf and swim. We have three healthy children and three healthy grandchildren.*** *I do cut down my consumption in the presence of my grandchildren. (a smoker who can't quit)*

*****

People need to be educated about the effects of tobacco; it's not a joke. ***It's not fair how one person's "habit" can ruin another person's health and ability to live their life the way they could and would like to.*** *(a lifelong nonsmoker)*

*****

During the last year two of my friends have died from throat and lung cancer caused by smoking. I was pretty close to one of these men and he was only forty-nine. Another guy I know here and consider a close acquaintance has recently had to have part of his throat and tongue removed because of smoke-induced throat cancer. Today, during a visit with my mother, I was told that my sister also has throat cancer, and my mother will go into the hospital next week for a test to determine if she has colon cancer. Whether or not this is related to her dipping snuff, I do not know. I have peptic ulcers and I'm told that my smoking is partially to blame and prevents them from healing, even though I'm on medication. (a smoker who can't quit)

*****

To be a tobacco smoker in today's society shows a complete disregard and disrespect for one's health. *I was a two- to three-pack-a-day smoker for over thirty years and did not heed the advice of anyone about the dangers of smoking. I smoked Camels and always enjoyed their tobacco; I didn't realize they added hundreds of other chemicals to their tobacco. I acted immaturely when people attempted to educate me about the potential hazards of smoking, not only to my own health but also to those around me exposed to my secondhand smoke. (a former smoker)*

*****

Two of my best friends who also smoke have been hospitalized for long-term care. Both have been denied patches or any help to combat their nicotine dependency and both have deteriorated mentally. Both have been medicated with Prozac. That is not the answer, but ***the medical world does not care about smokers.*** *(a smoker who can't quit)*

*****

I really would like to be free of the tyranny of tobacco; I'd like to be able to "take it or leave it." I can tell the damage smoking for more than fifty years has done to me. *I often have lung congestion, and when I awake in the middle of the night or early morning I cough up phlegm. My ability to walk fast is also impaired. Tobacco use will definitely affect my future. I have been* *a strong, robust person for most of my life. I felt like my body was good for more than ninety years, but if I can't stop smoking I'm afraid I might not get past seventy-five. I don't mind dying but I don't relish the thought of a painful, lingering illness before death. Also, I don't want to leave my wife a widow. I also worry about being hospitalized and not being able to smoke. (a smoker who can't quit)*

*****

I quit the second time when all the publicity about the danger of smoking hit the press. I was about sixty then and my brother had cancer. I gained almost fifty pounds and decided I would just as soon die from cancer as a stroke or heart attack. (a smoker who can't quit)

*****

My husband and I are both tobacco users and we lead a very active and physical life. We are much healthier than most people our age. ***Nonsmokers would have you believe all smokers are curled up in a fetal position with an oxygen mask from the age of twenty-five.*** *(an unrepentant smoker)*

*****

Another uncle died because of heart problems and throat cancer, both related to smoking. I had two friends die from throat cancer caused by smoking, an aunt who died from stomach cancer and an uncle who has it now. ***They all smoked heavily, although I'm not sure how much their smoking had to do with their cancer.*** *(a smoker who can't quit)*

*****

My husband, who never smoked or drank and ate all the right things, died last February of prostate cancer. He was seventy-four. He was exposed to cigarette smoke all his forty working years as a railroad trainer. The other men would come in the small cab to warm up and immediately light up; my poor husband had to inhale their second-hand smoke. He also inhaled fuel fumes from the engine. He exercised regularly. I know of no one who lived a cleaner, healthier life than he did, but he still died of cancer. (a lifelong nonsmoker)

*****

It bothers me when alcoholics or people who drink and drive tell me not to smoke because of the harm I am doing to myself. It bothers me when obese people give me the same advice. ***The people that I know who died of cancer never smoked a day in their life.*** *(a smoker who can't quit)*

*****

For most of my sixty-nine years I have been affected by tobacco—my father, other family members and coworkers smoked around me. *At a very early age (preschool) I began coughing night and day while inside the house. Doctors said I had "bronchial trouble" and would outgrow it. They said the night air was injurious to me and recommended cod liver oil and exposure to sunshine when possible. I coughed all through grammar school and high school, awaking each morning feeling tired and needing more sleep. I knew I was keeping Daddy awake—he needed rest and sleep before going to work. My brothers and sisters complained that I was keeping them awake. I became tense and worried, and that caused me to cough more. In public and to this very day, people have shoved Lifesavers, other hard candies and gum at me when I begin to cough. This has always bothered me because they do not help, even if you could suck or chew while coughing without aspirating them. People mean well, but more than sixty years of being reminded that your coughing is disturbing is a little much to cope with. (a lifelong nonsmoker)*

*****

I am getting frightened now because I feel smoking is beginning to affect my health. *I have chest discomfort, I'm short of breath, I get bronchitis frequently, and when I get a cold it hangs on for weeks. I always thought I'd quit before I was old. I used to hate to see old women smoking. Time flies; I'm now fifty-five. I look like an old smoker and I'm starting to be afraid I won't live long enough. I have a thirty-six-year-old daughter who is mildly retarded (I can't even think that smoking during my pregnancy was a contributing factor). She needs me.* ***A number of years ago my doctor asked me when I was going to quit smoking. I quipped, "Probably when it's too late." Now I'm afraid that will be a self-fulfilling prophecy.*** *(a smoker who can't quit)*

*****

Now that smoking is considered unacceptable, ***I feel quite guilty when I light up in front of someone. All it does is add to the list of things to feel guilty about, not to mention the fear of damage to my own health.*** *I wish there were some easy way to quit and get back to feeling like I did when I was a nonsmoker. I can discipline myself with other things in my life, but not smoking. (a smoker who can't quit)*

*****

I am weary. I've suffered more than sixty years of coughing from secondhand smoke; I'm tired of the embarrassment, of apologizing, of explaining, *"I don't have a cold. I'll not make you sick." I'm tired of the* *inconvenience, of the urinary incontinence caused by coughing, of coughing until I vomit in public, of losing sleep, of feeling tired, etc., etc., etc. (a lifelong nonsmoker)*

*****

I had a serious weight problem and my doctor recommended that I reach for a cigarette instead of food (can you believe that?). I tried but I was like a fish out of water. I didn't know what to do with the darn cigarette, and now I am glad, Glad, GLAD! (a former smoker)

*****

I am a happy tobacco user. I have smoked for fifteen years. I thoroughly enjoy it and don't want to quit. I know all of the risks involved. I see them in my family every day. Many of my family have died from cancer. My father was a smoker and died recently from congestive heart failure, and my mother was a smoker and is now having radiation for lung cancer. I knew all of the risks before I started. I started smoking by lighting cigarettes for my mother and sneaking puffs. I was a regular smoker at seventeen. (an unrepentant smoker)

*****

Two years ago I was hospitalized with a lung ailment. Because I smoke, the doctors immediately jumped to conclusions. When all the facts were in, the lung abscess was caused by the aspiration of foreign material during oral surgery. When I first entered the hospital of course I could not smoke. I went cold turkey. After three days the doctors agreed to start me on the patches. Immediately, when the nursing staff saw the patch order, they treated me very differently from how they treated me the first three days. I was furious. I had several nurses who would come in and say, "Oh, so you're a smoker, huh?" Immediately my defenses came up and I started to explain that what I had had nothing at all to do with smoking. They gave me everything from contemptuous to skeptical looks. After that I just said, "If you want to know my history, read my chart." Smokers were treated differently from the other patients; we faced everything from contempt to slow care. (a smoker who can't quit)

*****

Before my mother died of liver cancer in 1991, she kept bragging about how smoking had not gotten the best of her; cancer was totally unrelated to her smoking, in her opinion. Whether or not she really believed this, I'll never know. *One thing she did know was that smoking was bad for her. My mother had been a smoker for over fifty years, always bragging about her good health. Two weeks before Christmas, on her seventy-sixth birthday, she succumbed to cancer, which had spread to her liver before she ever realized she was* *ill. Since she chose to enroll in hospice upon learning of her illness, I became her full-time caretaker, on condition that she not smoke. She did stop smoking, but it was too late. Six weeks after learning of her illness, she died. (a lifelong nonsmoker)*

*****

Then, there is the medical profession. It is amazing what they can blame on a cigarette. You go to the dentist and hear the condescending, "You're a smoker, I see," and the eye doctors attribute vision problems to smoking. We are contemplating changing our family physician because he relates everything to our smoking. We can't get through an office visit without a "gentle reminder" to quit. Believe me, after I've been sitting in his waiting room for an hour, I don't need to be reminded that I want a smoke. The hospitals are another big irritant. The no-smoking policies are absolutely out of line. ***When a smoker is hospitalized, the addiction does not just disappear. It is real. It is physical. It needs to be addressed and dealt with.*** *Recently, one of my husband's coworkers was hurt while at work. He was taken to the hospital and had surgery on his hand. When my husband got off work, he asked me to take the guy a cigarette; he had been in the hospital for ten hours or so and was desperate. I went to the hospital and offered the smoke. Of course, the nurses were not pleased, but the guy wanted it bad enough to get out of bed and go down two floors to the outdoor sitting area—trailing his IV. The medical profession has got to acknowledge smokers' addictions. (a smoker who can't quit)*

Stories

Every Role Model I Can Recall Was a Smoker—A Former Smoker

I was born in 1932, the son of a registered nurse and an insurance salesman. My father abandoned us when I was four months old, leaving my mother a single parent long before this was socially acceptable. Because of this, teachers, administrators and my peer group singled me out for very unwanted attention. I saw my father only once; he visited briefly (ten minutes) when I was around five.

Both my single parent family status and an IQ above the ninety-ninth percentile set me apart from my peer group. I eagerly sought acceptance, but that was difficult to attain. In fact, until I reached full maturity I strove for peer acceptance in every way that I could in a futile attempt to appear "normal." I'm quite certain, at least in retrospect, that this was the underlying motivation for me to begin smoking at such an early and impressionable age and later to continue smoking. I took up smoking to "be one of the guys," enlisted in the Navy and volunteered for submarine duty. Subsequently, I re-enlisted, but this time in the Army; I was a tough, two-fisted sergeant. I have also worked as a high-iron worker, a construction boilermaker, a policeman and many other occupations—I performed quite capably in all of them.

Every role model that I can recall was a smoker. My mother remarried when I was twelve, and both my stepfather and his father—whom I particularly admired—were smokers. My parish priest and the bishop of our Episcopal Diocese smoked, as well as my physician, local politicians and community leaders, General Douglas Macarthur, President Franklin Delano Roosevelt, and my hero, John Wayne. One of my high school sports coaches was a chain-smoker, and I recall even now the obvious yellow stains on his fingers attesting to his cigarette habit.

Smoking was banned for students in grade school and high school, but understanding teachers (who were also addicts) observed this in the breach by not going out "behind the gym," or into the boys' toilet area where we smoked between each and every class.

I still have vivid memories of being sent into the teachers' lounge to deliver a message. The smoke was so thick that it was impossible to see who was in the room! Radio and infant-stage TV prominently featured cigarette advertising, and I can still recall the very repetitive jingles and slogans beamed at us at every commercial break like, "More doctors have switched to Camels than any other brand!" Wings cigarettes sold for ten cents a pack, and storekeepers universally ignored the law against selling to minor children. I can remember how my friends and I howled in protest when the price advanced to twelve cents a pack.

My stepfather bought Lucky Strike cigarettes by the carton. When I didn't have money to buy cigarettes—earned from lawn-mowing, caddying, working in a bowling alley—it was very convenient to filch a pack from his carton. While he told me that I couldn't smoke, I really don't know whether he actually didn't notice my petty theft, or whether he knew and was tolerant of it. I suspect the latter was the case.

I enlisted in the Navy two weeks after high-school graduation. I was seventeen. The cigarette companies advertised how they were doing their patriotic duty to "the boys in blue" by providing them with free cigarettes, which they did very generously. Later, "in the fleet," I was able to buy cigarettes from "Sea Stores" whenever we were out past the three-mile limit. They were seventy-five cents a carton initially and later up to a dollar a carton. When in port for extended periods we had to buy from the "Ship's Store," at approximately twice the "Sea Store" price.

A nonsmoker—I don't think we had one aboard—would have been extremely uncomfortable aboard our submarine; every man-jack smoked, from the captain down to the mess-cooks.

I began having severe sinus attacks when I was around twenty. Sailing submerged in a submarine with snorkel gear was often excruciating. Whenever seawater covered the valve that supplied breathing air and air for the huge diesel engines, it would slam shut and the engines would quickly draw a vacuum in the boat. As the engine man, I had to shut down the engines manually at a pre-determined reading on an altimeter. Typically, this would be at the equivalent of 18,000 feet of altitude, and it sure was tough on a sinus condition. It was a stupid and macho, but the engine men would compete to see who would wait longest to "chop" the throttle. A game of submarine chicken. We get "too soon old and too late smart."

At around thirty-five, I was having problems with bronchitis and pleurisy. I'd get one or the other, and sometimes both on the average of probably three or four times a year. In my late forties, I contracted pneumonia three different times.

By the time I was fifty-six, I had worked for many years as a construction boilermaker, and for a shorter period as a welder in a shipyard that built submarines. At both jobs, I worked closely with asbestos; I was almost buried in the stuff at times. I became informed (due to my eclectic reading habits) that I was at high risk for lung cancer because of the combination of asbestos exposure and cigarette smoking. This worried me, but not enough to quit smoking. I got a chest X-ray and cancer check-up every year. These showed nothing alarming, but my declining health resulted in the loss of my business. I filed for bankruptcy. I lost my fabricating business (twelve employees), my equipment and vehicles. We managed to hang on to our house, which also housed my wife's fledgling business.

Three months after my most recent X-ray, I stopped my car at a traffic signal 200 miles from home, coughed and spat a mouthful of bright red blood onto the pavement. Was I scared? You bet! Cutting my trip short, I drove home and made an appointment with my doctor for the very next day. He ordered chest X-rays and other tests. Two days later, he called me into his office and told me that he strongly suspected that I had lung cancer. It came as no surprise, but I still felt as though I'd been hit with a very large hammer.

The doctor told me that time was of the essence. He also warned me that the treatments to follow would be extremely expensive; he knew that I didn't have any health insurance. My best bet, he said, was to apply for treatment at the VA Hospital. The closest one with adequate treatment facilities for major surgery was 185 miles away. I checked in two days later and was quickly diagnosed with lung cancer. First, they would have to cure me of double pneumonia and get me strong enough to withstand surgery remove my entire left lung.

Ten days after what I call my "chain-saw surgery," a severe infection in the chest cavity necessitated opening me up again. This procedure is roughly akin to being hit by a speeding train; no one really expected me to survive. They were nearly correct—I hovered near death for several weeks. I spent seven weeks in intensive/critical care and a total of ten weeks in the hospital. Figuring that I would go home and die I checked myself out against doctors' advice. I am probably one of very few who has literally been able to see their own heart beating; the wound in my back had not healed at this point, and an interested observer could see my raw heart beating through the hole. Although my wife was trained to change the dressings at home, she found it too repugnant a job so a home nursing firm was contracted to handle this chore.

Just before the cancer diagnosis, my marriage had been very strained. I had established a small business for my wife as a hedge against the possibility that I might be incapacitated. I wanted her to have "a way to go" if I was unable to continue as our main support, or if we separated. The hospital was 185 miles from home, I was thought to be dying, and she had her business to maintain, which was her sole livelihood. She could only visit an average of twice a week. The feeling of abandonment was devastating! A very few friends made sporadic visits, but this was the loneliest period of my life.

During this time, most of my closest friends grieved my loss, even though I wasn't yet dead. They were embarrassed in my presence and didn't know what to say. After I recovered somewhat, they shunned me because subconsciously they felt that I had not done what I was supposed to, in spite of their having already wasted all that grief on my behalf. I don't see them anymore.

Recovery was slow. I have a degenerative joint disease, and that in itself is a disability. Realizing I desperately needed physical exercise if I was ever going to be more than wheelchair-bound, I decided to take the bull by the horns. I surveyed past physical activities that I had enjoyed, and compared the list with what I thought I was capable of performing and came up with canoeing. However, I learned quickly that I couldn't carry a relatively heavy canoe out of the water. Searching for alternatives, I found an ad for a fiberglass kayak that weighed only twenty-eight pounds. It was springtime, and I hadn't seen mountains in a long while, so I drove to the kayak factory in Kentucky, picked up my new boat and learned, on my own, how to car top it by myself. This little boat probably saved my life! It gave me an independent means of pursuing pleasurable physical exercise and gave me back a large measure of self-esteem. Although it wasn't designed for it, in about a year I was paddling in white water and boffing five-foot drops over waterfalls.

I need to add that six months after leaving the hospital, my wife and I agreed to separate; we divorced six months after that. After three years—I tend to date my recent life from "when I got out of the hospital"—I was stagnant and depressed. Then an ad caught my eye for classes for private detectives at the local tech school. I had nine years of experience as a policeman and several more as a deputy sheriff, so I reasoned that this class would be an interesting way for me to get out of the house and meet people. It certainly met my expectations. My prior police experience qualified me to take the detective agency examination, and the next thing I knew I had a license hanging on the wall. I achieved the highest score that has been posted in the past fifteen years.

I never intended to leave retirement and go back to work, but I found that perhaps it was possible to do so, and it sure beats watching the boob tube! It's stimulating, and I love it! I have also returned to magazine writing freelance when the gumshoe business is slow.

Now, five and a half years after surgery, my ribs still hurt like hell. The doctors told me that they had to be broken during surgery, and were not set like they should be. "When you're feeling better, come on back in, and we'll re-break them and re-set them properly." Yeah, right. Don't hold a bed open just for me.

My endurance is very limited, and I tire easily because one lung can't do the work of two. My body cries for better oxygenation, and I can get out of breath over a game of chess. Also, sex is really challenging, and my partner always wonders if she should call 911. I can walk a quarter mile in summer heat, but really need air conditioning to help me breathe with less tiring effort. Climbing stairs is daunting. However, I have conditioned myself to do things that almost seem impossible, like kayaking.

Smoking appeared desirable and sophisticated during my impressionable and formative years, and about all of my role models and peers smoked. It was also very accessible, and it was inexpensive enough to be enabling. I know it damn near killed me. On the other hand, I have little patience with people who blame "Them" or "Society," or "Life," or "The Devil," etc. for their misfortunes. My personal philosophy is to take charge of my life and thus take responsibility for all that befalls me, although my ego must surely suffer.

I am certain that, although I have been "cured" of cancer, my life expectancy has been significantly reduced. The normal life expectancy for healthy, white males is currently seventy-two years and here I am sixty-one already and realistically, not "healthy." Tobacco use has exacted a big toll from my life and no doubt shortened what remains of it.

More Than Likely I Will Not See My Grandchildren Grow Up—A Former Smoker

My story really begins when my mother was diagnosed with throat cancer, and later died from kidney failure. When my close friend at work then died from cancer of the lungs, I began to get scared and realized what I was doing to myself and probably had done to my family over the years.

My fear grew stronger when I was diagnosed with chronic bronchitis. The doctor said that I should quit now before I developed emphysema, which he said could be as bad or worse than cancer, because it has no cure and more than likely would kill me.

My breathing problems and my ability to do things got worse. Two years later I was diagnosed with emphysema. I take four different medicines to help me breathe and to make me sleep.

I worked through this time until July, when my doctor told me I would have to quit work. I was using three times as much oxygen to go from Point A to Point B as someone who did the same thing at a run. Half of my breathing was just wasted energy; my lungs no longer would absorb oxygen the way that they should. The last time I saw my pulmonologist, five months later, he upgraded my emphysema to severe chronic obstruction pulmonary disorder (COPD).

Although I've been through pulmonary rehabilitation, I still have these fears deep down inside: Will I wake up in the morning? Will I wake up gasping for air, as I have done before? Or, perhaps I will have a severe breathing attack, burst blood vessels and drown in my own blood. Perhaps I will have a heart attack from the immense fear growing inside every day.

You live with this terrible disease, which is slowly but surely killing you, and there is very little you can do but take medicines and realize it's going to catch up with you sooner or later. You know you're going to miss a lot of the wonderful things in this life because you screwed up for a stupid thing like a cigarette.

I'm still fighting this disease and probably will fight until I become a burden to others, at which time I will quit fighting. At first, I thought I was tough and could handle it. But I'm not as tough as I thought. I would ask my doctor questions, pray when I was alone. I even prayed for death at times. More than anyone else, my wife has been my greatest support.

I can see the results of all my years of smoking in my family. More than likely I will not see my grandchildren grow up. I will not be able to play games with them as I have always looked forward to doing. Smoking has also affected my life with my children. They have taken so long to realize that I'm really this sick. I still have my doubts that they totally believe I am this sick. Smoking affects my life with my wife in personal and other ways, but she is a very understanding human being, probably more than the average. She is a registered nurse; she knows more about how to deal with the sickness and realizes what I have ahead of me.

I realized I was addicted when I tried to quit so many times unsuccessfully. Whenever I would try to quit, I would feel like something was missing. I needed the weed just to cope with life. It is only when you get away from it that you realize you don't need it, that it was a total waste of your money and life.

I tried many times to quit without success after my mother died. Her death made me want to quit and I did after many attempts. I think the biggest hurdle was convincing myself that I had to quit. Once I had completely convinced myself, I was able to do it and lost the desire to smoke altogether. I quit when I actually realized I was killing myself. Along with millions of other smokers, I was killing myself making the tobacco industry rich.

I first tried smoking when I was in fifth grade, at about eleven or twelve. My cousin was there and tried it at the same time. I actually started smoking regularly after my sixteenth birthday. My mother had told me not to, but for some reason, I did it anyway. Today I'm very sorry for disregarding her advice, which was not like me, as my mother and I were quite close.

I guess I continued smoking because there was a lot of peer pressure to smoke, and I really didn't think it would hurt me. When I started smoking it was not considered bad—most guys smoked. I actually felt I enjoyed it. Now I believe it was the addictive aspect of the drug I enjoyed, I just never had enough sense to quit. It really felt relaxing after a meal and seemed to take the edge off my nerves. This should have been a clear sign of my addiction.

My Doctor Told My Husband I Was a Human Time Bomb—A Former Smoker

My husband and I started smoking in our teens—he at sixteen, me at eighteen. I started because he smoked; he started because his friends smoked. We are now seventy-one and sixty-seven. He smoked regularly for fifty years; I smoked for forty-five years.

The addiction is frightful. As anyone who has been a smoker knows, the habit builds and builds. I started with two or three cigarettes a day; when I finally quit four years ago, I was smoking over one-and-a-half packs per day.

In the sixties, my doctor tried and tried to get me to stop, but like everyone else, I rationalized. I reasoned that it wasn't cigarettes, but rather car exhaust fumes that caused illness. We lived near Los Angeles at the time, and the smog and exhaust fumes were terrible. My husband and I quit smoking once for seven months, but were unable to quit permanently. When we went back to smoking, we smoked more than ever. My husband began to believe smoking was unhealthy, but he could not give it up.

In 1990 we moved to Hawaii, where we lived our golden years. Two years later, my husband was stricken with lung cancer; they excised the smallest cancer they had ever seen and thought they got it all. He quit smoking immediately on hearing the news.

I continued to smoke for another two years outside the house and away from him, until my doctor insisted I take a stress test. An angiogram was ordered and I was told to go home and not get up for anything until the date of the procedure. My doctor told my husband I was a human time bomb. I continued to smoke! I had no pain, so I was sure the doctors were mistaken. The angiogram was scheduled for 2 p.m. in Honolulu, and I was on the operating table at 6 p.m. the day before Thanksgiving for double bypass surgery.

I stopped smoking ten minutes before the angiogram. After the bypass surgery, I was in ICU for eight days. When I returned home, it was very difficult to continue to abstain from smoking. It was hardest after eating, when talking on the telephone, or when enjoying a cup of coffee or cocktail. Now that I'm smoke free I wonder why I ever enjoyed it, but I really did. I cannot stand the smell of cigarette smoke now.

My husband had a recurrence of his cancer, and so there was a second operation. The cancer had not metastasized. This time they removed the top lobe of the right lung. It took almost a year for him to recuperate. The next year cancer cells began to grow in the rest of the lung and so there was a third surgery—they removed the entire right lung. Eight months later, the cancer had entered the trachea, and he had to have five weeks of radiation. The Cancer Society helped with hotel accommodations, but it was still an expensive experience. It is now eight months later, and although he feels better than he has felt for some time, a CAT scan reveals something in his liver.

This has devastated our lives. If only we had known what terrible destruction smoking could cause. But, someone does know: all the doctors, politicians, and cigarette manufacturers. Why does our government continue to subsidize tobacco farmers and then pay Medicare for all these terrible bills? Why can't there be a class action suit against the cigarette manufacturers? Maybe that would wake the public up to the dangers of tobacco. Stopping the advertising was just a slap on the wrist.

The doctors say that smoking did cause my husband's problems as well as my own! Is anybody listening?

It's Not Fair How One Person's Habit Can Ruin Another Person's Health—A Lifelong Nonsmoker

I am allergic to cigarette smoke. I blame the job I worked at for seven years for my current health problems. I worked in a smoking office where they allowed smoking in the downstairs break room. There was no outside air exchange and the smoke from the break room was re-circulated through the ventilation system and throughout the entire office building. You could tell the minute someone went on break or when there were meetings downstairs as the smell was immediately circulated upstairs. In the summer I would open the window in my office and put in a tiny fan to bring fresh air in, but in the winter the windows would freeze shut so it was more difficult to get fresh air.

About seven months after I started the position I got earaches, my equilibrium was off, and I had a consistent sore throat. I went to the doctor continuously for three months; he said he couldn't find anything wrong with me. Finally, he said I did have an inner ear infection and treated me with antibiotics—the symptoms did lessen for awhile. Then, I started getting more and worse colds, even in the summer, which I had never experienced before. In winter it seemed I was always sick and even got bronchitis after my colds and sinus infections.

After I'd been there five years I started seeing the doctor frequently again. I was experiencing sore throats, sinus headaches, and earaches within two hours of going to work. Yet on the weekends, my symptoms would disappear. I started experimenting by taking sick time and vacation time Thursdays and Fridays when I felt really sick; my symptoms would disappear within a day away from work. When I entered stores or restaurants or encountered someone who was smoking, my symptoms would reappear. By Thursday I was so run down, I could hardly force myself to get up and go to work. It was a chore to get through the last two days of the week.

My doctor finally gave me some nasal spray and pills that cost me $100 a month. They helped, but there were steroids in the nasal spray so I wasn't too happy about being on that or any other medication for an extended period of time. My doctor also told me that if they weren't willing to do something about the situation at work I should look for another job. My body had become so run down that if I did get seriously sick I be able to fight much off, and if I continued to subject myself to the situation I was in I could end up with serious health complications as I got older.

They rearranged the office and my desk ended up no more than three feet from where everyone hung their coats. My symptoms worsened when smokers would hang their coats up. I finally asked that they remove the coats from my office. They were, but it was a big joke around the office with the smokers and even the upper management. They had been informed of my medical problems and knew of my doctor visits, but it was like no one believed me. It seemed that they thought I was just causing problems.

Finally, they decided to remodel the entire office. In the blueprints of the remodeled office layout, I would be moved out of my current office with a window and placed in an area without a window. My only air exchange would be two vents that re-circulated smoke from the break room. I asked if they could relocate my office to the corner by a window or at least have a ceiling fan put in above me; I got no comment on either request.

I went to my doctor and he again said that I needed to do something myself if my employer wasn't willing to. I asked him if he could write a letter to my employer explaining my medical problems and asking them to consider giving me an office with a window as I felt they weren't taking me seriously. He did and I gave it to my supervisor. I was asked point blank why I was trying to cause problems. I was told I was not a team player and that I should probably find a different job since I was unhappy. I wasn't invited out to lunch or drinks after work with coworkers anymore. And, for the first time in seven years, I didn't get my yearly raise. Everyone avoided me.

I continued to do my job as well and there were no negative statements made when I had my yearly review. I also started looking for other job opportunities in a smoke-free environment. I was fired for "not being a team player" two weeks after they received my doctor's letter. I've had two part-time jobs since the full-time one, but I had to leave each even though they were in smoke-free offices because their ventilation systems were hooked up to other offices that were not smoke-free.

My life is no longer normal. I avoid restaurants, bars and public places where I may encounter smokers. Even if someone is driving down the road smoking and I come up behind them, I can tell right away; in the grocery line I can point out the smokers immediately. I have been looking for work I can do out of my home.

This is how cigarettes and secondhand smoke have affected my life. People need to be educated about the effects of tobacco; it's not a joke. It's not fair how one person's "habit" can ruin another person's health and ability to live their life the way they could and would like to.

I'm Fighting the Entire Courthouse Over Smoking—A Lifelong Nonsmoker

My name is Jackie and I work as a deputy clerk at the county courthouse in an eastern tobacco-growing state. Most people around here call me Jobetta, from Job in the Bible. I have never been a smoker myself, but I have worked around smoke all my adult life. I have been a deputy clerk for nineteen years. I didn't realize what working around all the smoke was doing to me until about five years ago when I began experiencing severe respiratory problems. I was diagnosed with respiratory allergies to pollen, dust, and mold. Exposure to cigarette smoke all day at work aggravated my respiratory problems, and this went on for two years. I finally asked my allergist to write a brief letter to my employer explaining this. He agreed and wrote a letter explaining my situation, concluding with: "Any assistance you can provide to assist her in establishing medically acceptable working conditions will be appreciated."

I asked my employer to ban smoking from the workplace. I felt it was not really fair to force me from my job because of what other people were doing to me while they smoked. Besides, I couldn't afford not to work. I continued to suffer breathing problems throughout the winter. I began to have chronic pain in my chest from allergies and asthma. The doctor at the pain control clinic wrote to my employer:

> I am seeing Ms. J H in my clinic. She has chronic refractory pain in the left thorax that I believe is being significantly worsened by working in a smoke-filled environment. I would strongly recommend that some dispensation be made for her work environment and that she be afforded a no-smoking area for her to work. I believe that this situation is significantly worsening her pre-existing medical condition, and she would show good improvement if this were remedied.

I continued to petition my employer for smoke-free working conditions. By this time many public buildings were beginning to have designated smoking areas. The federal government had banned smoking in federal office buildings except in designated smoking areas, but these federal protections did not apply to the state level. The courthouse was scheduled for renovation; it was a convenient time for my employer to consider putting in the renovation plans some designated smoking areas away from where my coworkers and I worked all day. The problem was that current state laws restricting smoking applied only to schools and penitentiaries. My employer didn't have to do anything to improve working conditions, and so didn't, that is, until…

The governor of our state issued an emergency regulation ordering agency heads to implement "a reasonable smoking policy in state-owned and occupied buildings." The order was to continue to allow smoking in state buildings, but only in designated areas. Exactly where the designated areas would be was left up to each agency head, but the order stated that "Employee suggestions and complaints shall be considered when designating smoking- and nonsmoking-areas." Best of all, for me, the order stated clearly that "No employee shall be involuntarily assigned to a work station which has been designated a smoking area."

I immediately requested that my work area be clearly marked a no-smoking area. I asked my doctor again if he would write to my employer in support of my request. He wrote:

> This is to certify that JH is a patient of mine suffering from severe bronchial asthma, chronic allergic bronchitis, and chronic obstructive airway disease as well as allergic rhinitis, allergic rhinosinusitis, and migraine headaches.
>
> Because of her exposure at work to cigarette smoke and coal fumes, and because there is no ventilation in her work area, she has had severe symptoms of coughing, wheezing, shortness of breath and severe headaches. This has caused great loss of work time as well as infirmity. The patient has been unable to sleep because of the severe coughing and has not been able to function normally because of the above described exposures and conditions.
>
> We would appreciate it if you could do something to clear up this situation in her environment in order to allow her to work adequately and live a more normal life.
>
> Your cooperation will be greatly appreciated and if you desire any further information, please let us know.
>
> Sincerely yours,
> LDM, M.D.

I was overly optimistic. Though none of my coworkers' smoke, many of the people who came to the office for driver's licenses smoked heavily. Even though the governor's order urged agencies to install ventilation in smoking areas to remove the smoke, our office is not ventilated and nothing was done to prevent people from smoking in our presence. Although my doctor had suspected coal fumes as part of my problem, in the summer when the heating had been off for several months, my asthma attacks became more frequent and intense. I would have difficulty breathing; I would wheeze and had a terrible dry cough at work. I would feel better after a weekend away from the office. No one in my home smoked. My husband had quit smoking nine years ago. My medical bills climbed. The local doctor referred me to specialists at the university medical center. I was put on five different asthma medications. The university doctors wrote to my employer describing my medical condition, pleading with them to provide an environment free of tobacco smoke.

In the winter, after I had been to my doctor on almost a weekly basis for over three months, my doctor wrote my employer the following:

> Mrs. H. has a history of having problems with respiratory allergies that have been exacerbated during the fall and winter, being exposed to excessive cigarette smoke in the courthouse. This extreme exposure has caused her numerous medical problems including exacerbation of her asthma and her breathing difficulties. It has been my recommendation to her to avoid such cigarette smoke as this can cause worsening of her asthmatic condition, and can also lead, by chronic exposure to second-hand smoke, to lung cancer.

It's been five years and I have not stopped pleading. This summer I asked my doctor to write to my employer yet again, and he did. It's not just for me, I am sure there are many others like me that work in the courthouse who have allergies and other health problems that are severely aggravated by the smoke. The smoke in the courthouse is not only hard on courthouse employees; in the nineteen years I have worked here I have heard many, many complaints about the smoke-filled condition of the courthouse. I think that I am speaking for ninety percent of the citizens of this county when I say it would be wonderful to walk into the county courthouse and not come out gasping for breath. The Surgeon General has already proved the health hazards of secondhand smoke.

My health has deteriorated and my medical bills are mounting—our insurance is not very good either, I have found out. I am fighting the entire courthouse over smoking. I have been trying for several years to get a local ordinance passed to stop smoking in all workplaces, with no luck. I contacted OSHA a year or so ago, but they told me there wasn't anything they could do until some laws were changed—that's all I hear from everyone.

I can't afford to quit my job, or to be without insurance. This November, my doctors wrote one more letter to my employer. The letter stated my medical history and the fact that I was on nine different medications for respiratory problems. The letter concluded:

> The most disabling problem Ms. JH has that I follow here at the clinic is her recurrent pneumonitis and bronchitis. She has multiple allergies and due to smoke-filled environment where she works she has recurrent asthmatic bronchitis-type episodes and requires frequent hospitalizations and clinic treatments for this condition. In my opinion, from the above medical conditions and examinations of Ms. JH and on her recent examination in my office I find her to be completely and totally disabled and unable to do any type of gainful employment at the present time.

I would rather keep on fighting than take disability retirement. I made the choice not to smoke myself, yet I have been disabled by other people's smoke. I just recently filed a worker's comp case trying to get somebody's attention higher up than here. I have seen a doctor almost every day for the last six weeks and my body is wearing out rapidly. I really believe without my strong faith in God I would be in heaven now. As you can tell, I don't give up easily.

I Initially Thought of Smokers and Dippers as Villains, But Have Come to Think of Them as Victims—A Lifelong Nonsmoker

The issue of tobacco is a complex and emotional one for me because of both personal and professional experiences. I was born and raised in "tobacco country," eastern Northern Carolina. As far back as I can remember, most adults I knew smoked: Aunts and uncles as well as my parents. I knew cigarette brands, package and billboard images and TV jingles by heart at an early age, and it seemed that every major movie and TV star smoked or advertised cigarettes. Before church, the men would stand outside smoking and talking. Exiting after the service, they would immediately light up before making for their cars. I remember my parents telling me as I grew older that smoking wasn't good, that it would "stunt your growth, limit your wind," and so on; however, no one talked about it being fatal.

My favorite uncle kept a Camel pack in his shirt pocket at all times, had cartons sitting in his bedroom and ashtrays filled with butts. He said he couldn't quit smoking even though he coughed a lot. He was one who would have literally walked a mile for a Camel. Ironically, he threw his beloved Camels in the trash, never to smoke again, the day he was diagnosed with terminal laryngeal cancer. He wasted away and died a terrible, slow death in a nursing facility in his late fifties; it was 1964, the same year the first Surgeon General's report became public. Sadly, the report meant little to my family; most of them were fervent supporters of the local tobacco growers and powerful manufacturing cartels.

Coughing was the most memorable noise at family get-togethers. My brothers, cousins and I often suffered respiratory and sinus infections, but no one ever connected our exposure to smoke to these frequent and often-expensive nuisance illnesses. When aunts and uncles came over for adult card games, they played in a literal haze, the proverbial smoke-filled room. We kids sat observing, passively smoking right along with them. As I got older I realized that I didn't like being around smoke. It stank and stuck to clothes and hair. I knew that anything that burned my throat and eyes and made me cough couldn't be healthy, regardless of the cigarette advertisements to the contrary. Too many of my friends of youth smoked—many of them beginning in elementary school—falling into the trap of "being cool, grown up." Even the best athletes among them smoked with abandon, believing themselves infallible. We all thought we would stay young and healthy forever. Fortunately, I never fell into that trap myself, probably because I was exposed to so much smoking. I knew it was more noxious than appealing.

While in high school I began to hear medical news about smoking. I vividly remember the actor who portrayed the district attorney on Perry Mason appearing in a TV public service commercial begging people not to smoke; he was dying of lung cancer. Even though he was a regular in an aunt's favorite TV show, his appeal didn't work with her; she smoked till she died of ruptured aortic aneurysm in her early sixties. Another uncle had a heart attack in his mid-thirties. He too ignored the warning to quit smoking. I heard how his brothers sneaked cigarettes up to his room in the hospital where he stayed for six weeks; this was not uncommon in the 1960s. He eventually recovered, smoking all the while. I hounded him for years to quit. To this day, in his early seventies, he still smokes occasionally "for pleasure." He did quit his two-pack-a-day habit/addiction years ago, however.

His younger brother, another of my favorite uncles, a man who really "had it all," smoked every chance he got. We would sit together watching football games on TV while he filled the nearby ashtray. He carried a cigarette in his mouth always, even fishing. Even though he was a gifted and handsome athlete, I remember his progressive shortness of breath, even in his thirties. He ascribed it to "getting older," and blamed his premature wrinkles on too much sun. His addictive personality was manifested by his uncontrollable urge for tobacco and alcohol. He had several near misses in his early forties with alcoholic encephalopathy, mild myocardial infarction, and severe hypertension. He finally died an old man at the age of forty-eight from a massive heart attack that I believe was largely caused by the suffocating and toxic effects of his tobacco smoke. He succumbed to the "great cigarette deals" he got on his visits to North Carolina, when he and his wife would literally fill the auto trunk with cartons of cigarettes at such "great prices" because of low taxes and good old North Carolina's promotion of tobacco.

Other family experiences come to mind. An aunt died in her sixties three years ago after spending the last six months of her life in a nursing home, mindless from carcinoma to the brain from her beloved cigarettes. Before falling ill, she refused to visit relatives or friends who didn't allow smoking in their homes. This included a daughter she loved dearly; her addiction was stronger than her love. I remember her comment, "I'd rather die than quit smoking; I love it so much." She had no affection for anti-smoking activists, and I learned to keep quiet around her for fear of setting off a battle I couldn't win. She said they could all go to hell. Well, they are still around working for health and life, and she's gone—another RJR or Philip Morris soldier killed by friendly fire.

My father smoked Lucky Strikes "LSMFT," I remember saying as a child. I worked on him for years to quit, and he finally did before his untimely death in a work-related accident at fifty-five. My mom tried to quit for years, finally succeeding in the later years of her life. She died at sixty from heart failure. We still do not know if the damage was done before she actually quit; certainly, the smoking did not help her diabetic condition.

Many more family members died directly or indirectly from smoking-related illnesses. My maternal grandfather had lung and colon cancer. He coughed and smoked on his deathbed, his belly incision causing great pain, but not enough to obviate his smoking. Other aunts had various malignancies, some of which may indeed have been brought about by their two-pack-or-more-a-day smoking habit. My brother smokes to this day despite my attempts to encourage or cajole him into quitting. He knows as I do that his smoking will cause him illness and ultimate death if he does not stop.

Several cousins smoke and they complain chronically of allergies, respiratory infections and kids with ear and sinus infections. Recently, my favorite cousin called to tell me about an early Christmas present: he and his wife had quit smoking. I was elated for them and myself. He knew that he couldn't have given me a more coveted gift. Now I can invite them to spend time with my family and me without worrying about offending them by asking them to smoke outside. More importantly, I am relieved that I may be spared having to attend to another prematurely dying loved one and wondering at his funeral what more could I have done to prevent his death.

Even more personal, my wife of nearly twenty years smoked when I met her as a college freshman. She took up the habit in "self defense" because of the prevalence of smoking females in her dorm. She was one of few nonsmoking girls, even in 1970, and gave into be one of the gang. After meeting me in midyear, she struggled to quit smoking, knowing how I felt about the habit. I made it clear that I couldn't stand smoke and what it had the potential to do to her. Despite having smoked for only a few months, she still found it exceedingly difficult to quit, especially because of her smoking dorm-mates. Thankfully, she did succeed, and today is a fervent anti-tobacco activist.

I struggled with environmental tobacco smoke in my dorm and on campus at a time when smoking restrictions were nonexistent. My roommate smoked, as did several buddies; I sought a nonsmoking roommate after midyear and never allowed myself to be forced into that situation again.

Sadly, my family and I still suffer from forced exposure to tobacco smoke whenever we eat out, shop or attend certain athletic or entertainment events. We have progressively limited our activities because of this. Although I have voiced my complaints and recommendations as a nonsmoking citizen, my sentiments and us nonsmokers are not well received in this tobacco-money and tobacco-disease endemic environment.

The local producers, manufacturers, supporters, and economic beneficiaries are vehement and vociferous in their allegiance to tobacco; there is little recourse for health advocates. Local and state government agents and representatives are almost all tobacco allies, giving them at least lip service for tobacco-related votes and political contributions. Tobacco manufacturers, who have seemingly unlimited financial resources to sway public and political opinion, vigorously oppose anti-smoking ordinances. Their cronies in state government use whatever means necessary, including legislation, to promote tobacco and weaken anti-smoking and childhood smoking-prevention initiatives. The former lieutenant governor chaired a panel on youth drug abuse and refused to address tobacco use and its link to addiction in any way. To a person, our state representatives in the US Congress are staunch tobacco supporters. Our senators are tobacco champions. With many formidable foes of tobacco control, there seems little that nonsmokers and other health and children advocates can do.

When contemporaries fall ill or die, we are reminded of our mortality. I was shocked to learn of a childhood friend's lung cancer at the age of thirty-six. He had smoked since his early teens. He learned of his diagnosis after months of fatigue, weight loss and worsening cough. After the initial disbelief and regret, he underwent partial lung resection and follow up therapy, which was debilitating in itself. He partially lost his voice because of the location of his tumor; he can only talk in whispers. Mercifully, he seems to have been spared a recurrence and is otherwise doing well and enjoying his second chance with his wife and three sons. He has no desire to smoke again.

From a professional viewpoint, tobacco has had a profound effect on me as well. I encountered elderly and middle-aged victims of tobacco abuse while still a student at Bowman Gray School of Medicine, in the tobacco capital of North Carolina, Winston-Salem. We used to joke about RJR giving us both cancer research money and cancer patients. While people lay suffering and dying, undergoing biopsies, surgery, radiation, and other painful indignities too numerous to count, across town RJR conducted business as usual, a good business at that. We were bombarded with advertising on billboards along every major thoroughfare telling of company tours to proudly display cigarette manufacture, showing virile young "smokers" having a sexy good time using their products and describing the incredibly satisfying taste of their big name brands. Finally, by government mandate, a "warning sign" appeared, relegated to a small corner of the otherwise enormous and colorful advertisement, meaningless in the total context, laughable to the tobacco corporate and ad agency people.

At medical student bull sessions, especially after rotating through oncology, pulmonary medicine or autopsy service, we decried the billboard and glossy magazine ads as siren calls to the young, the next generation of good tobacco customers. As I learned of the myriad ways tobacco use inflicts injury and contributes to premature death, I became more incensed at the cynicism and hypocrisy of the entire tobacco industry.

I initially thought smokers, dippers, and chewers were villains, especially when I was subjected to their smoke and became aware of the enormous financial burden their health care, lost productivity, and prolonged dying lays on all of us. I now think of them as victims instead. They have fallen victim, however naively, ignorantly or stupidly to the ingenious ploys of tobacco promoters and pushers. Once hooked, and this occurs easily and quickly, many users cannot find the will or ability to quit, even unto death. I have seen so many patients embrace their own grim reaper in the form of a cigarette, even as it takes their lives a little each day.

During residency training in diagnostic radiology, I attended and learned from many patients who had smoking-related vascular, pulmonary, or malignant diseases. I performed arteriograms, biopsies, and innumerable other procedures in their diagnostic workups and therapy. There was never any billboard glamor, beauty or sexiness in any of it; I remember pain, fear, anxiety, blood, and waste. Entering private practice was another tobacco-related challenge. The radiologist I joined was a true tobacco addict, smoking upwards of four to five packs a day. I avoided being trapped in the same room with him as much as possible, but it was still very unpleasant and a source of contention. Patients complained of the smoke in the department, especially those individuals there for asthma, pneumonia, emphysema, and other respiratory complaints.

Although they were in the minority, back then the smokers held sway on the hospital board, on staff among the nurses and on the hospital floors. Very ill nonsmoking patients had to share their rooms with smokers until the Joint Commission of the American Hospital Association finally addressed the situation—they mandated smoke-free hospital environments. It was about that time that my partner retired. His forceful personality would never have allowed him the "indignity" of going outside to smoke. He believed it was his right to smoke when and where he wanted. His love of tobacco was manifest in his resigning membership in the American Medical Association when it issued a policy statement opposing tobacco use, recognizing it as a major public health threat and the number one preventable cause of early death and disability. Sadly, my partner paid for his loyalty with his life; he had a stroke shortly after retiring. He made a remarkable, though incomplete, recovery with intensive and expensive rehabilitation. Within five years, his lung cancer was diagnosed as inoperable. He suffered through chemotherapy until he found it intolerable. A massive heart attack spared him any further ordeal shortly after discontinuing the therapy.

A forty-five-year-old male patient once came through the emergency room with a fractured arm bone, his radius, from picking up a watermelon. His X-ray showed the break through a lesion in the bone, a metastasis from his lung cancer. I went into talk with him, asking if he knew he had cancer. He said he learned of it at another hospital months before; he had had surgery and thought he was cured. He had quit smoking. I had to inform him it was back, the cause of his pathologic fracture. He told me he had been smoking since he was thirteen. He said he knew smoking was bad and could cause cancer, but he said those famous words that have stuck with me, "I didn't think it would happen to me."

Another, a lady of about sixty, with severe chronic emphysema requiring continuous oxygen therapy, had a mass on her chest X-ray fairly classic for carcinoma. When the technician went to fetch her from the floor for her lung biopsy, she found her smoking in bed with oxygen prongs in her nose. After the biopsy, the patient asked my opinion of the diagnosis. I tried to be upbeat though we both knew the truth. She left saying, "I've decided to stop smoking." I didn't tell her there was no need.

A man in his early sixties, looking like he was in his eighties, also came in for a procedure. As he moved onto the table, he gasped for breath; his emphysema and chronic bronchitis smothered him whenever he exerted himself even slightly. I asked how he got by. He said he kept his oxygen close, slept with it and just didn't do much. I asked if he had smoked much in the past. He said he still did, that he needed a cigarette first thing in the morning to "clear his lungs" and that smoking didn't have anything to do with his lung disease anyway. He had gotten that way from working in a West Virginia coal mine years before. I realized argument would accomplish nothing, but stated my disagreement and encouraged him to try to kick his addiction. He left believing cigarettes blameless; if alive today, I'm sure he continues to smoke.

The hardest part of watching someone who is sick or dying from tobacco use is knowing that the illness and progression to death were preventable, that the horror of tobacco-induced illness and death was self-inflicted, caused by a loved one who smoked or was an occupational hazard of being chronically exposed to environmental tobacco smoke at work.

I continue to encourage friends, patients and acquaintances to stop smoking. Some avoid me and all my proselytizing; others humor me. I have actually had some success with a few. Some patients have come back to me to say that my concern and encouragement helped in their victory over tobacco addiction. I have written letters to the editor of my local newspaper, resulting in a storm of protest from the tobacco proponents, including invitations to get out of town and ply my trade in an area of more like-minded individuals, such as Boston. I may as well have attacked Mom, the Flag and Apple Pie. Letters to my representatives usually go unanswered or result in a brief reproach.

I'm Quite Weary of 60-Plus Years of Coughing and Secondhand Smoke—A Nonsmoker

Early in May of this year my sixty-four-year-old sister (one of five girls and two boys in the family) died of lung cancer. She had smoked for forty years. When she was diagnosed last July, the cancer had metastasized to her liver and bloodstream; she was given three months to live. She went to her doctor because she was short of breath. The diagnosis devastated us. I did not want her to die before me; I didn't want to give her up. She was the first of our siblings to die.

Mother is ninety and in a nursing home. My sister decided that she was not to be told of her illness or death. I've had mixed feelings about this, but respected Ruth's wishes. Ruth donated her body to medical science, which I've also had some difficulty dealing with; yet, I know her spirit is not there.

Ruth had quit smoking (cold turkey) three years before her initial illness. From the time she was diagnosed with cancer in July until March, she and her husband, a nonsmoker, visited my husband and me once a week for the day and dinner at a seafood restaurant. We played cards and had a good time. By March, she had developed three brain tumors and a tumor in her lung. Up until this, she had received no treatment, but at this time, radiation was used to shrink the brain tumors for her comfort. She was still on her feet most of the day and doing household chores. I would cook up food for her to take home. By spring, we would go to her house, fifty miles away, to bring food, visit and take her to the doctor.

I'm next to the oldest of seven children, so in a sense the five younger than I are like my children because my older sister and I cared for them when we were all young. I am sixty-nine. Our father smoked or chewed tobacco and died at sixty-two from a massive myocardial infarction following bilateral femoral bypass surgery.

For most of my sixty-nine years, I have been affected by tobacco—my father, other family members and coworkers smoked around me. At a very early age (preschool) I began coughing night and day while inside the house. Doctors said I had "bronchial trouble" and would outgrow it. They said the night air was injurious to me and recommended cod liver oil and exposure to sunshine when possible. I coughed all through grammar school and high school, awaking each morning feeling tired and needing more sleep. I knew I was keeping daddy awake—he needed rest and sleep before going to work. My brothers and sisters complained that I was keeping them awake. I became tense and worried, and that caused me to cough more. In public and to this very day, people have shoved Lifesavers, other hard candies and gum at me when I begin to cough. This has always bothered me because they do not help, even if you could suck or chew while coughing without aspirating them. People mean well, but more than sixty years of being reminded that your coughing is disturbing is a little much to cope with.

In school, I became very hot due to nervousness about my coughing, and the hotter I became, the more I coughed. It has always been very disturbing to draw attention to myself by coughing, especially in church. In all my adult life, whenever possible, I've removed myself from situations where I'd have to breathe cigarette smoke; however, that has not always been possible. I've also had to put up with a lot of tobacco smoke from hospital patients, nurses and doctors; it was only after my retirement that they banned smoking in our hospital. There were times while attending nurse meetings that I had to sit with my eyes closed because the smoke hurt them. Often my eyes would water and my nose would run as if I had a cold. On one occasion, I had a surgeon tell me he didn't want me to nurse his patient because he thought I had a cold.

In my adult life personal physicians have attempted to help me by prescribing antihistamines and cough preparations, but even they didn't fully understand my problem. From childhood, I always sang in church choirs, duets, trios, and quartets—when not coughing. Then four years ago my respiratory problem became so acute that I could not stop coughing and could not sound a note even after my cough improved. I would stand in church services and try to sing but not be able to make a sound, tears streaming down my cheeks. This has been very painful. Now I cannot hold a whole note or sing an entire line before I run out of breath. I've spent much and wasted a lot of time and energy going through tests and X-rays, and trying medications and treatments that have only made my life more miserable because of dreadful side effects. They have not improved my condition.

Because tobacco smoke is everywhere I go, I cannot enjoy the many events I'd like to enjoy in my golden years. I cannot even spend a night at the home of my daughter or son because both my son and son-in-law smoke. I cannot breathe too well after visiting there during the day and have to go outside frequently. When they visit my home, they go outside to smoke. My two young grandchildren want us to spend Christmas Eve and Christmas Day with them. In order to do this, I have to have cough syrup with codeine, which is difficult to get. My internist and my allergy specialist will not prescribe it because they are afraid of addiction. Also, due to the drug abuse in our society, the narcotic records of doctors and pharmacists are examined regularly. Whenever I ask at the pharmacy to sign for a preparation with codeine I'm very uncomfortable doing so and I don't like the treatment I get when I'm out of my home territory. They simply say, "I don't have any!"

I am weary. I've suffered more than sixty years of coughing from secondhand smoke; I'm tired of the embarrassment, of apologizing, of explaining, "I don't have a cold. I'll not make you sick," of the inconvenience, of the urinary incontinence caused by coughing, of coughing until I vomit in public, of losing sleep, of feeling tired, etc., etc., etc.

CHAPTER 7

Lifestyle: The Power of Tobacco Over Our Lives

For both smokers and nonsmokers, tobacco can determine one's daily activities, livelihood, relationships, and health. Tobacco can determine matters from as important as keeping or losing one's job to matters as trivial as deciding where to have lunch. If one is allergic or addicted, the entire day's routine, indeed, one's whole life must take into account this fact: A chronic smoker cannot leave the house without her cigarettes and lighter and can only go where she will be able to smoke; a nonsmoker with severe allergies must also plan his daily activities to avoid exposure to smoke and other irritants.

Control is a central issue here for many smokers and nonsmokers. Nonsmokers, particularly those with severe allergies and other respiratory problems, often feel that smokers deprive them of control over their lives, livelihood, and health. This is especially true of nonsmokers whose lifelong exposure to smoke has deteriorated their health to the extent that they live in fear of encountering smoke. These nonsmokers, including smokers who have quit, report that smokers and secondhand smoke have become a major determining factor in their lives. Many feel robbed of their health and the chance to live carefree lives.

Many smokers also feel that they have lost their autonomy, admitting that the addiction to tobacco rules their lives. Tobacco becomes part of one's lifestyle: Smokers who attempt to quit have a difficult time adjusting to a routine without a cigarette in hand because the rituals of smoking become part of every minute of one's day. For many smokers, the cigarette is a necessary part of each meal, conversation, cup of coffee, or

I. Newman and J. DeFrain, *Tobacco Use and Intimate Relationships*,
https://doi.org/10.1007/978-3-319-92579-0_7

cocktail; the workday, including breaks, is impossible without cigarettes, as are moments of stress and times to relax. What initially seems to be an enjoyable accessory to the routines of daily life inevitably becomes a necessity: The cigarette becomes central.

Many relationships have been constructed or destroyed around tobacco. Smokers and nonsmokers tend to avoid striking up or maintaining friendships or acquaintances with each other. Both sides admit a sense of social ostracism because of their relationship to tobacco: Smokers feel they are targets of discrimination and abuse, and assertive nonsmokers feel that because of their "extreme" positions on tobacco, they too are isolated and silenced. Because many smokers and nonsmokers avoid each other in social and other situations, both groups cultivate unrealistic stereotypes of each other. For example, smokers seem to feel that they are more sociable and friendly in comparison with nonsmokers, while nonsmokers cultivate a perception of smokers as generally obnoxious and inconsiderate.

Obviously, seeing any group of people as an indistinct and homogenous population only adds to the problems of tobacco use. However, dialogue is possible though difficult, as many smokers have loved ones who don't smoke, and vice versa. Additionally, former smokers are a potential medium for the beginnings of constructive dialogue, having experienced the problems of addiction as both smokers and nonsmokers. For both smokers and nonsmokers to take back control of their lifestyles, dialogue is essential.

Testimony

I got along well with my coworkers and had many friends, including three who were very close to me, but I could almost never join them for lunch or a drink after work even though I would have loved to. Once, when I was reassured that this one restaurant had excellent accommodations for nonsmokers, I very hesitatingly agreed to go. Well, it had been years since I laughed so much; I had such a great time! I drank nothing but soda and coffee, but I was so exhilarated I felt like I was "high." ***That night, it came crashing down on me—all that I'd missed for so many years. I've had allergies since I was nine and my social life was on "life support" by the time I got to high school, since most of my friends smoked. I was not consciously aware of it, but I was going out less and less.*** *(a lifelong nonsmoker)*

*****

We also have found ourselves limiting whom we invite to our house for an evening or a meal. Rather than not smoking, we just don't invite nonsmokers. *We have many friends who don't smoke and I find that I never invite them over. If they do just "drop in," we try to reduce our smoking or make sure we sit in a well-ventilated area. It is always a problem. (a smoker who can't quit)*

*****

Traveling has become more difficult. Whenever possible, I stay in all smoke-free hotels. *When this is not possible, I always inspect the "nonsmoking" room to make sure it is not surrounded by smoking rooms and that it has not just been converted from a smoking room. I rent nonsmoking cars, and inspect them before renting. My husband refers to it all as the sniff test. I go to the grocery store at my destination and cook my own food. When driving long distances, I carry my own food in the car; it is so difficult to be guaranteed smoke-free dining on the road. I spend so much less eating out now, due to the scarcity of completely smoke-free restaurants, especially the expensive ones I used to frequent. (a lifelong nonsmoker)*

*****

It makes me angry that I let smoking control me. I thought this was one thing in my life that I controlled – how wrong I was. *(a smoker who can't quit)*

*****

I am highly allergic to tobacco smoke and have had many a meal ruined by the secondhand smoke of the unfortunate nicotine addicts who also frequent restaurants and public places. ***Just going out can and does frequently make me ill. Yes, even in restaurants with so-called separate "smoking sections," as if smoke is not ubiquitous.*** *(a lifelong nonsmoker)*

*****

Smoking has definitely affected my social life. I have turned down invitations to homes and parties where I knew there would be no opportunity to smoke. *I will go if I know the duration will be two to three hours, and decline if I know it will be longer, knowing I will be miserable without a cigarette.* ***I have not made friends with nonsmokers I would like to be friends with, avoiding potential problems before they can occur.*** *(a smoker who can't quit)*

*****

Sometimes avoiding smoke was impossible in order to socialize, such as attending football games and dances. *The heavier the smoke, the more difficult I found it to breathe. At dances in smoky rooms, I would have trouble dancing—ending up gasping for air. I would have to stop and find a way to gracefully leave or go hide out somewhere until I could breathe again. I looked for ways of staying out as much as possible when I went home on semester breaks.* ***I hated returning to the smoke in my parents' home.*** *(a lifelong nonsmoker)*

*****

On our tenth anniversary at an elegant seafood restaurant, I took Tupperware containers along knowing I would have to pack up my lobster dinner and make a quick getaway when the smoke got too bad for me. *It embarrassed my husband when I placed the Tupperware on the table next to my champagne glass, but I was just trying to inject some humor into the situation. We stopped going to restaurants at all, except at a local, hamburger-counter truck stop, the only local place we knew that didn't allow smoking. (a lifelong nonsmoker)*

*****

My spouse smokes. ***Our friends are opposed to our smoking and to smoking in general; therefore, I can't be with them for long without leaving them to go out for a smoke. This puts a damper on friendships.*** *(a smoker who can't quit)*

*****

I harbor a great deal of anger toward the tobacco drug dealers. Anger over the effects of tobacco use on my life colors a great deal of my thinking; tobacco has greatly influenced how I have been allowed to lead my life. *Tobacco was for many years more important to my parents than me. Even today when I have trouble breathing, I cannot go where I want to go or do what I like. I feel as though I have spent my whole life on the outside looking in because of the tobacco industry's greed. (a lifelong nonsmoker)*

*****

Asthma impacts where I can eat, who I can carpool with, whose invitation I can accept to visit their home. *I am a teacher, and this is the first year that we have a smoke-free school. It is wonderful! Before this year I had to avoid smoking areas and smokers who still carry the smell on them. (a lifelong nonsmoker)*

*****

Since reaching thirty-five, I've organized my life to omit smokers. This means that my social contacts are mainly limited to those who are nonsmokers. *I avoid all social gatherings where smoking is allowed. The effects of other people's smoke have always clouded my enjoyment of movies and other public events. Now, in California and other places, smoke-free public places have greatly helped me enjoy life. There still remains the fact that even if one chooses to eat at an outdoor facility, smokers may still be upwind of your space and therefore render your meal only marginally enjoyable. (a lifelong nonsmoker)*

*****

Although I have always been opposed to smoking, I have stopped tolerating it since my mother's death. *I no longer go dancing because there is virtually no place to go that is smoke-free. Gambling casinos will never get my money (they got a lot of my mother's) so long as they remain giant ashtrays.* ***It is astounding how little entertainment is available to people who will not tolerate smoking. Almost all night life is out of the question. You have to be much more inventive, do most things in the daytime, and engage in much healthier forms of entertainment.*** *(a lifelong nonsmoker)*

*****

Within the last three weeks, I have been diagnosed with a medical problem that may require surgery and have been told to quit smoking. I'm not sure which I fear more, quitting or surgery. My whole adult life has revolved around smoking. Every habit, relationship, crisis, decision, lifestyle choice has revolved around smoking. Cigarettes have been my "best friend" and my worst enemy. *Cigarettes are my stress outlet, my calming mechanism, my stimulant and my relaxant. They are part of everything I do every day from getting up in the morning to sleeping at night. I have attempted quitting three times, once successfully for three weeks. I returned though because I want to be a smoker more than I want to be a nonsmoker. I don't know myself as a nonsmoker and don't know that I want to. Today, however, I'm not sure what I want. As I was telling a friend recently, I don't think I've ever been more afraid in my life. I told my doctor I would need more than just a patch to quit smoking. I don't know what I'll do. I stand at a major crossroads. I truly wish I had never started smoking. I ache for the teenagers I see start every day. I wish cigarettes were illegal—and no longer available. (a smoker who can't quit)*

*****

It's very strange that as a smoker I couldn't imagine a life of not smoking. *If I entered a building I would note whether or not they allowed smoking, and if not I had to figure out how I could get out of there and when, in order to smoke.* ***As a nonsmoker for fourteen months I can't imagine a life of smoking—everything tastes and smells better. I don't have to worry if I have matches, tobacco or pipe. When I was smoking I went through a constant ritual, patting each of my pockets to make sure I had everything I needed to smoke with every time I went out.*** *(a former smoker)*

*****

I cannot work in any environment where smoking is allowed. This limits my ability to seek and obtain employment and has hampered my career. *In the past I have gone on job interviews where the interviewer was a smoker several times. I became physically ill at these interviews. Sometimes the interviewer would smoke during the interview. Other times, the office was permeated with smoke even if the interviewer was not smoking at the time of the interview. In several cases, I turned down job offers due to the smoking environment, and was not offered jobs after telling interviewers I needed a nonsmoking environment. (a lifelong nonsmoker)*

*****

During all this time my social life was very limited. Spontaneity went out the window. Any invitation to friends' or relatives' homes had to be refused if there would be any smokers there. *Sometimes smokers would refrain or go outside if weather permitted, but there was always tension and embarrassment, and often hostility. I was a member of Parents without Partners for several years. The only activities I attended were theater outings and the occasional outdoor event. Restaurants were a problem, as well as dances and weddings. They still are. I lost some friends, and had to give up seeing very much of my closest (geographically) relatives (an uncle and his wife who live near Toronto). However, I did adapt to this period of social isolation, and was pleased when smoking became more and more socially unacceptable. I did quite well for a few years, changing my lifestyle completely to one of eating nutritious foods, avoiding foods identified as allergens, and trying to avoid chemicals and perfume as much as possible. (a former smoker)*

*****

I won't lie; it has not been easy to be so intolerant of such a widespread habit that many regard as a constitutional, or God-given right. I've lost friends, a good part of my social life, missed family gatherings, and angered a lot of people in public places. *My lifestyle on a daily basis could be considered very boring and dull. No matter where I go, I always have to* *consider whether smoking is permitted. If more nonsmokers would stop tolerating smoking in their presence, I am sure that society would turn around on this issue and nonsmokers would be able to go anywhere we wanted. Most nonsmokers seem to feel guilty for restricting smokers—as though they are restricting a child and punishing him or her by doing so. Smokers are childish; they have to do what they want, whenever and wherever they feel like it, regardless of the consequences. But they are the ones restricting our lives, punishing and torturing us with their cancer sticks. They pollute our air, our lungs, our hair, clothes, buildings, and cars with their smoke. It is an addiction, a slow form of suicide, and they don't seem satisfied unless they can take a substantial number of nonsmokers to the grave with them. Why do nonsmokers put up with this nonsense? If somebody ran around in public pointing a loaded gun at their head, and kept turning it on other people as well, they would quickly be arrested, or worse. A cigarette is no different than this loaded gun. Lit, it is loaded and pointed at everyone around. Yet, as a society we ignore this, passing watered down anti-smoking ordinances with countless exceptions, and then not enforcing them. (a lifelong nonsmoker)*

Stories

"Why Should I See a Psychiatrist to Learn to Accept Inhaling Toxins and Carcinogens?" I Asked—A Nonsmoker

It all started while I was still in college. My father was a plumber and was up by five in the morning; he had to be at work by seven. At first, when he started with that horrible coughing, which would wake me up in terror, I thought, "Oh, he's not going to work today—not with that cold." After weeks and months went by, the fear set in as I realized that it was no cold.

While I was still in college, he was diagnosed with bronchitis, which later developed into chronic asthmatic bronchitis. By this time, he was retired. His "smoker's cough" sounded more like retching, but came only occasionally thanks to medication and an inhaler, which he used six times a day. At this point, things were okay; the coughing and throat clearing were only a mild annoyance. Four or five years later, dad was diagnosed with emphysema. Goodbye to his beloved bowling—his only distraction, hobby, and social life. His attacks scared the life out of me. Watching him suffer like that often brought me to tears. He could no longer lift or carry more than four or five pounds of anything. Two years on, at sixty-nine, my father was diagnosed with advanced, large-cell lung cancer.

At this point, my dislike of cigarettes and smoking mutated into pure and absolute hatred. I read everything I could get my hands on: the effects of secondhand smoke; about laboratory rats who, given a choice between nicotine and food, chose to starve; about radiation particles; and how chemicals in cigarette smoke include rat poison (arsenic), insecticide (acetonitrile), explosives (ammonia), the lethal agent used for capital punishment (hydrogen cyanide), rocket fuel, and antifreeze (methanol). I learned that by definition, nicotine is an alkaloid poison, and that if someone were to inhale in a single dose the amount of nicotine in merely one pack of cigarettes, they would die.

They were all set to do radiation treatments on my father when they discovered that the cancer had metastasized to the bone; they started chemotherapy. It was working and we were cautiously optimistic. Unfortunately, it lowered dad's white blood cell count and they discontinued that treatment after his second bout with pneumonia in December. His second chemotherapy lasted five hours once a month. Dad only got sick once, and then not too badly. He would be tired for several hours after the treatments. But my heart was breaking and I was starting to lose hope. My father was always a quiet, reticent man; he was happy just to read the paper, watch the birds out the window and enjoy a few favorite TV shows. Up until now, I'd never had a real conversation with him, but now he wanted to talk, and I wanted to listen. It wasn't much, just about the "old days" and stuff like that, but it was precious to me. I could not and cannot understand his acceptance of his disease; for him, it was there—end of story. He had no "rage against the dying of the light." But I raged.

They discontinued the second chemotherapy. His third and final treatment was simple enough: a hypodermic at the doctor's, and then one pill a day for five days after the shot. Well, the shot went fine, and on the next day, he took his first pill. One hour later, it was as if someone had hit him over the head with a hammer. In one stroke, he became a desperately ill man. It struck me hard. Although he had chronic asthmatic bronchitis, emphysema, and lung cancer, I was never able to think of my father as "sick." Silly, isn't it? He couldn't even make it down the three steps to go outside, and except for hospital stays, he was housebound. This was November 1986.

By the first two weeks of March the next year, he was dying. His body, wracked with cancer, was shutting down fast. On the morning of March 17, my mother woke me up to help her move him. (Mom had a stroke, six month s before dad was diagnosed with cancer. She had surgery and went into cardiac arrest the day after her operation.) I could hear the fluid gurgling in my father's lungs as he fought to breathe; he was drowning in it. The ambulance took him at 10:25 a.m. We were at the hospital most of the day. He died peacefully, so they told us, at 10:30 that night shortly after a morphine injection.

After my father's death, to an outsider, even my friends, I was no more "militant" about smoking than before. Inwardly I raged. I could never bring myself to be angry at my father for causing his own death because he was my father, and partly because I sympathize with people who started smoking before there were warnings on cigarette packages about the dangers of smoking. In my less rational moods, a part of me feels that my father committed slow suicide. Smokers have a death wish or they delude themselves about the harmlessness of tobacco. With my father's death, something in me cracked. My world was pulled out from under me and I lost pieces of myself; I will never be the same.

I said I wasn't angry with Dad, but I did rage. I couldn't see anyone smoking without silently wishing cancer on them. After all, they were asking, begging to be given cancer! Fortunately, that feeling soon mellowed into, "My God, what the hell is wrong with you? Don't you know what you're doing to yourself?" Well, I'm mostly—not completely—past that now, though if I were given the word "cigarette" in a word association test, I would definitely respond, "cancer." Cigarettes and cancer are Siamese twins, in a sense, one and the same. Though I'm not as bad as I was that first year after dad died, I flatly refuse to inhale cigarette smoke. I don't look for confrontation—I hate confrontation, but not as much as I hate cigarettes.

My social life became nonexistent. I simply refused to inhale all those carcinogens and poisons. What sane person would act otherwise? Sure, we have an air pollution problem in New York, but being in a closed-in, unventilated room with several smokers exposes you to so many more poisons and carcinogens than a walk down Fifth Avenue. Besides, transportation and manufacturing are necessities and serve a common good, while smoking is merely an individual pleasure.

In the past fifteen years, I've been to a restaurant less than ten times. Twice, I've walked out in the middle of a meal because I couldn't take the smoke anymore. For years I didn't set foot inside a movie theater. At Lincoln Center and Carnegie Hall, I stayed in my seat or walked up and down the aisle at intermission because I couldn't take the smoke outside the seating area. I felt like a pariah.

Three years after my dad died I was interviewing for a job and asked my soon-to-be boss about the smoking policy, explaining that I couldn't tolerate cigarette smoke. She told me there was no smoking allowed anywhere. County law forbids smoking in open areas, and the whole office was open. I told her I didn't mean to cause any trouble, but I found the office quite smoky. She went to the office manager and the owner, and both said that within a week there would be no smoking. I should've smelled a rat, but took all three at their word. After months of fans, smokeless ashtrays, and having to leave work early—without pay—I finally wrote an intelligent, calm, and informative letter to the owner of the suite stating that I was promised at the interview that there would be no smoking, but that this had not yet come to pass. They called a meeting. One smoker went ballistic and the owner threatened to destroy my boss's lease. In the end, smoking was really banned.

I got along well with my coworkers and had many friends, including three who were very close to me, but I could almost never join them for lunch or a drink after work even though I would have loved to. Once, when I was reassured that this one restaurant had excellent accommodations for nonsmokers, I very hesitatingly agreed to go. Well, it had been years since I laughed so much; I had such a great time! I drank nothing but soda and coffee, but I was so exhilarated I felt like I was "high."

That night, it came crashing down on me—all that I'd missed for so many years. I've had allergies since I was nine and my social life was on "life support" by the time I got to high school, since most of my friends smoked. I was not consciously aware of it, but I was going out less and less. But college was great! I majored in music. I virtually lived in the music building! And, for whatever reason, almost no one smoked. I had tons of friends and things were great; it was the best time of my life. All my difficulties began when I started working after graduation. The building I worked in was sealed, and the ventilation was often turned off to save money.

A coworker once told me I needed a psychiatrist because I asked him, politely, to smoke elsewhere. (I had to be in the files that day, there were plenty of places for him to move to, and I offered to help him move his stuff.) I thought about what he said; I fully realize that part of my aversion to smoking stems from my perception of smoke and that it isn't totally due to my allergies. But WHY SHOULD I SEE A PSYCHIATRIST TO LEARN TO ACCEPT INHALING TOXINS AND CARCINOGENS?

At least I can go to the movies and some restaurants now because of New York City's smoking regulations; however, more often than not they're ignored and the Health Department doesn't have the resources to keep up with all the complaints.

My current "philosophy" is "hate the smoke, respect the smoker." I have some degree of sympathy for smokers because I know they're addicted to a drug more addictive than cocaine, heroin, or anything else. It still makes me angry that the amino acid tryptophan was taken off the market because a few dozen people died due to a single tainted batch, but it's just fine and dandy that 450,000 smokers and an estimated 53,000 nonsmokers die every year because of cigarettes. It's damned scary what the tobacco industry can accomplish with money and power. I love America, but it is obvious that if you have money and power, truth be damned!

Four years after taking the job I quit because I was moved to an office where "smoke-free" was understood to mean "smoke freely." That is the distance I will go to avoid inhaling secondhand smoke; I just won't do it. Some people think I'm nuts. I know it's extreme, but is it wrong just because it's not what most people do? I see a day far in the future when people will wonder how their ancestors could've been stupid enough to roll poisonous leaves into paper, burn, and suck the resultant smoke into their lungs, knowing that chances are one in three that they will die. In Poe's time, less than 200 years ago, mothers would put wads of opium in their baby's mouths to make them stop crying. Now we cringe at the thought. Someday, we'll cringe at the idea of smoking.

My Whole Existence Was Just to Endure Each Working Day and Go Home—A Nonsmoker

I grew up in a home where both my parents smoked fairly heavily. Back then, in the 1940s and 1950s, I never heard people speak of tobacco smoke as a respiratory irritant, but I knew that I greatly disliked tobacco smoke; it made breathing difficult for me. I hated the smell of the house when I got home from school every day. When I was little my parents had card parties with their friends all smoking in the living room; I would lie in my bedroom just waiting for them to all leave. I particularly hated having to use the bathroom Sunday mornings after my mother had spent an hour smoking continuously in the bathroom while preparing for church. After my father added a small bathroom and shower off my parent's master bedroom, I asked permission to use his shower instead of my mother's bathroom, but I didn't tell him it was because of the smoky smell in the other bathroom. I just told him I liked the shower better.

My father smoked a pipe occasionally. I used to smell his cherry pipe tobacco in the humidor sometimes because I sort of liked its smell, but not the smoke. My mother always smoked when she was driving. Her smoke made it hard for me to breathe in the car when she drove me to piano lessons or other places. I asked her once not to smoke while I was sitting next to her because it bothered me; she became angry with me and said I was making it up. I would have to sit with my face turned out the car window to try to get fresh air and to avoid breathing her smoke.

When I was about ten, I was diagnosed with asthma. I was hospitalized for several days because of asthma and was unable to attend the last few weeks of the fifth grade. I took my exams at home and later was bedridden most of one summer because of asthma. Most physical activity, such as skipping rope, running, going out in night air, participation in school sports, gym, and dancing, was limited. In high school, I was in drill team one year, but my lungs always hurt. We did not have the inhaler medications then that we have now, and I regularly went to the doctor's office for injections of theophylline and sometimes cortisone. The family doctor told my parents I was probably allergic to feather pillows and oranges, and that I would outgrow my asthma.

The last summer before college I refused to go on our family's two-week summer vacation because I didn't want to be in the car with my parents smoking. My parents were upset at my refusal to go, so I let them think it was because I preferred to keep working at my summer job.

I started college in 1962. My first dorm roommate asked if I smoked. When I said no, she offered not to smoke in our bedroom, an unexpected kindness, and one that, in retrospect, still amazes me. I hardly ever socialized in the dorm lobby or watched television in the dorm rec room where people smoked; I also avoided spending time in the rooms of dorm mates who smoked in their rooms, even if they were friends. Consequently, I was fairly solitary. My mother encouraged me to smoke; she had learned to smoke in college because so many of her friends smoked. I once bought a pack of Salem Menthols, locked myself in my dorm room and tried to learn to smoke. I thought that getting used to it was just a matter of mind over body, then I wouldn't mind being around acquaintances and friends who smoked. Within seconds, I was choking. I opened the window and fanned the horrible smoke out.

Sometimes avoiding smoke was impossible in order to socialize, such as attending football games and dances. The heavier the smoke, the more difficult I found it to breathe. At dances in smoky rooms, I would have trouble dancing—ending up gasping for air. I would have to stop and find a way to gracefully leave or go hide out and somewhere until I could breathe again. I looked for ways of staying out as much as possible when I went home on semester breaks. I hated returning to the smoke in my parents' home.

At my first temporary job at an aerospace plant, smoking was only allowed in restrooms, so it didn't bother me much during the workday. My first full-time job at an insurance company was in a huge room of about thirty desks. I don't recall seeing people smoke all the time—there was still a modicum of proper business behavior, but some people smoked during coffee breaks at their desks, and there was always a faint odor of smoke in the room. When someone lit up at a desk near mine, my throat would catch and my nose would hurt.

I started having frequent colds and upper respiratory infections during my two years at this job, but I didn't make the connection to smoke. Once, when I mentioned to my father my dislike of smoke at work, he admonished me to get used to it if I wanted to get along with people. Years later when my father himself had stopped smoking because he believed the first Surgeon General's report, he still tried to discourage me from openly complaining about smoke, even after I became really ill.

A few of my old college friends, whom I still saw occasionally, smoked around me, but I didn't ask them not to because I was afraid of alienating them, and because I figured I could put up with the occasional smoking. I don't recall dating men who smoked, or perhaps they just didn't smoke around me. When I met my husband, we each felt that we couldn't have become serious with or married someone who smoked.

The last year at my first job, there was a clerical worker across from me who smoked from the time she arrived at her desk until the end of the day. She would leave her burning cigarette in her ashtray with the smoke drifting right in my face. The smoke would trigger sharp pain in my sinuses, sneezing, runny nose, itchy, watery eyes, and headaches. Since I had no choice but to face her while working (because of the placement of our desks and typewriters), I asked if she could point her cigarette away from me so that the smoke didn't blow in my face. Not only did she refuse, she was indignant at my request. Later, she started eating in the very small employee lounge where I regularly ate lunch; fifteen minutes into lunch she would light up and start blowing smoke in my face across the dinette table.

My husband Stanley and I were married in a small ceremony at his parents' home. A few of the guests—my mother, an aunt, and an uncle—smoked in the dining room during the reception, even though we had asked them not to. Throughout our married life, Stan and I have avoided socializing with, maintaining friendships with, or inviting into our home people who smoked around us. At our first apartment, I seldom sat around the swimming pool or patio because so many people smoked there. When friends invite us over, we explain that because of my asthma I can't attend if there is going to be smoke. I can only recall one instance when a hostess accommodated me by requesting guests not to smoke in her house. At my insistence, Stan often attends parties or wedding receptions without me because I don't want people to think that he is antisocial as well. We didn't go to movie theaters for many years until smoking was restricted there. In restaurants, we asked for nonsmoking seating, but because there was still smoke in the air, often we ate quickly or left without finishing our meal.

A few months ago at a regular gathering of acquaintances in a restaurant, Stan's host refused to sit in the nonsmoking section because his wife wanted to smoke; now Stan no longer joins their get-togethers. On vacations over the years, we have sneaked hot plates, toaster ovens, or microwaves into our motel rooms so that we wouldn't have to eat out in smoky restaurants. We have been stranded and starving on vacations trying to find a smoke-free restaurant, and ending up having to buy food at a market.

Once we rented an apartment by the ocean, where we had requested nonsmoking accommodations. The room smelled fresh when we walked into it late the first night because the manager had left all the windows open wide and it was freezing with fog and the cold ocean air. However, after we went to bed, I awoke with asthma and ended up trying to sleep in the car. It ruined our entire trip because we couldn't find another place to stay.

Later, we started imposing on relatives from time to time because they didn't smoke and had some extra space. We used to go ballroom dancing when we were first married, but eventually stopped because I couldn't take the smoke in public ballrooms and because my asthma got too bad for me to dance. We loved attending Dixieland music concerts at pizza parlors and monthly gatherings, but stopped going years ago because of the smoke. Even classical music concerts without smoke were difficult to find, so eventually we started attending the happy revival of classical music performances in church settings where smoking is not permitted.

In about 1972, I transferred jobs to a different branch of the district attorney's office for the County of Los Angeles. A number of employees smoked in the office, not just at coffee breaks but throughout the day. One lady with whom I became friends used to smoke as she sat by my desk to talk until I told her the smoke bothered me. After that, she refrained from smoking near me in the office or when we went out socializing. People who conducted business in our office took chairs right next to our desks and smoked right in our faces for long stretches of time every day. I asked them not to smoke next to me, but they would just move about three feet away and continue smoking.

My respiratory symptoms increased after two or three years in this very smoky atmosphere. When I could no longer sleep at night and my symptoms had become fairly chronic, I went to an allergist who diagnosed asthma and chronic severe rhinitis, sinusitis, and pharyngitis. After taking my medical history and doing allergy tests, the doctor had no doubt that I was having a reaction to smoke. He offered to write a letter to my employer saying I needed to work in a nonsmoking environment, but I was embarrassed about it; I felt that smoke was just something I would have to tolerate as long as I worked. I did tell my clerical supervisor (an occasional smoker) about my health problems due to smoke at work, and she very nicely designated the clerical room under her jurisdiction as nonsmoking. Of course, the rest of the office suite and hallways were still smoky. Fifteen years later, when I asked her for an affidavit for one of my legal cases, she clearly recalled that "You were obviously suffering and not able to breathe."

In 1979, I transferred to another branch of the district attorney's office closer to our home in the Valley. When I interviewed for this job, I thought the office was fairly smoke-free. As it turned out, the heaviest smoker was absent and the others in court the day I interviewed. When I began work, there was smoke drifting right into my face from an attorney's office a few feet away from my desk. Several other staff members smoked whenever they were not in court, as did a secretary whose desk was behind mine. I was still taking allergy shots and other medications, but within a few months my asthma became worse. I tried to avoid going into the offices of smokers.

I asked the attorney who smoked all day a few feet from my desk if he would shut his office door; he said I could get up and shut it if I wanted. I was up and down shutting that door constantly because he would come and go, and others were in and out of his office all the time. The secretary who smoked behind me was nice when I explained my problem to her, and she began stepping out of the clerical room and down the hall to smoke. Of course, the hallways, law library, stock room, reception office, restrooms, and lunchroom all smelled of smoke.

Because of escalating asthma symptoms, I was sent to the hospital emergency room twice, and once I was admitted for several days' observation. My asthma always improved away from the smoke, whether at home, in the clean air of the doctor's office or in the hospital. Finally, my allergist wrote a letter to my employer saying that because of my asthma I needed to work in a smoke-free environment. When I showed the letter to my supervisor and asked her if she could help me by at least restricting smoking in the clerical room and getting smokers to close their office doors, my supervisor said "You can ask people if you want to." Then, my supervisor began smoking at her desk during her lunch hour. Before that I had never even seen her smoke, and she had always gone home for lunch.

I started seeing a pulmonary specialist who put me on medication for about a year or more to try to control my asthma. I tried to find other methods to help myself; I practiced deep breathing exercises and meditation and took walks that got slower and more difficult as my asthma worsened. I attended a self-help group for asthmatics. I tried to become more tolerant.

In 1983, a new supervisor moved to the desk next to mine; she chain-smoked. A few hours after her arrival, I started having choking spasms, couldn't breathe, coughed uncontrollably, my eyes welled up, and I was gasping for air. I went to the ladies' room where I fell to the floor crying, trying to breathe. Finally, I threw cold water on my face until I stopped gasping and choking. I tried to go back to my desk, but because of all the smoke my throat started closing up again and I had to leave the room. I was homesick with asthma for the next two days. My doctor put me back on medication and wrote another letter to my employer recommending a smoke-free work environment for me. When I returned to work, I asked my new supervisor if she would mind taking her smoke breaks somewhere outside of the clerical room, or if she would let me move to a desk in another room. She angrily refused.

I appealed to her superior, also a smoker, and gave him my doctor's letter. He shoved the letter back at me and said, "There was someone in another office who complained too much about the smoke, and the county took care of him all right. If you don't like it, get out!" I felt like I couldn't go on, and after talking to my doctor about it I filed for worker's compensation. The next day I received a threatening phone call from another superior who said if I didn't show up at 8 a.m. the next morning, whether I was sick or not (I was at homesick with asthma), he would personally see that I was fired. I asked my union for help, but they refused to become involved; at that time, there was no county policy on workplace smoking.

I needed to work, we were just starting to pay a lengthy mortgage on a house, and I couldn't jeopardize my income. When I arrived at work the next day, the level of smoke throughout the office and hallways was greater than any time before. I was so sick I could hardly walk across a room because my breathing was so bad. I could hardly talk on the phone. Another superior from the district attorney's office had come to see if I showed up at 8 a.m. He told me that if I was that sick I shouldn't even be there, even though my own superior had threatened to fire me if I failed to return to work. I felt not only physically ill, but persecuted. To add to the harassment, another attorney with whom I worked took me aside and said he had been delegated to "deal with" me. He said the county didn't like my assertive attitude about the smoke, and that they would do anything to get rid of me now. He said he would help me keep my job if I would withdraw my worker's compensation claim. Under such duress, I did so.

During this time, I had also been calling around the county looking for a transfer, but because my legal clerical job was unique to the district attorney's office, I would have had to take almost a fifty-percent pay cut to accept a clerical job in another department. Also, none of the other county departments had smoke-free environments either, so I would have gained nothing by the transfer. After writing a letter asking to have my personnel file purged of any records pertaining to my smoking complaints, and after putting in writing that the matter was being handled internally, I was allowed to move to a desk in a small reception passageway a few feet up the hallway from the smoky clerical room. It was enough improvement that I was able to keep working, even though my asthma remained only barely tolerable.

The only office computer at that time was next to my smoking supervisor's desk in the clerical room where I used to work. The supervisor required me to spend two hours or more a day working at the computer, during which time she smoked with her cigarette right next to my chair. I asked her if just for the two hours I was there, she would mind smoking somewhere else. She started sitting at my desk in the reception area to smoke then, so that when I finished at the computer and returned to my own desk, my room smelled of heavy smoke. When I asked her if she would smoke somewhere other than my desk, she said it was the only place comfortable for her, so I would have to choose between her smoking at my desk or smoking next to me at the computer.

In 1985, the county enacted a nonsmoking policy that on its face purported to guarantee any employee the right to a smoke-free work environment; however, there was only minimal or superficial change in the smoky conditions of the office.

I put in a work requisition to have the air-conditioning filters checked and was told by the serviceman that ninety percent of the circulating air came from outside and there wasn't any smoke in the air. I still asked to have the air tested for smoke content; a judge in the courtroom on the other side of the wall from the district attorney's office had complained about smelling smoke in his courtroom and had the air tested there. When I asked my boss, he told me to get the hell out of his office and go file a grievance. Other coworkers and some secretaries I had been friends with for a long time also hated the smoke, but they were afraid to say anything. An attorney who was slightly asthmatic complained repeatedly about the smoke to the boss. When she presented him with a letter from herself and a few other attorneys who wanted the nonsmoking policy better enforced, they were told not to expect career advancement unless they withdrew their complaints.

I wrote a letter to the attorney heading a committee for improving the quality of the work environment in the district attorney's office; I asked him to help get better enforcement of the nonsmoking policy. He did not acknowledge my request. Someone brought in a large portable air filter for the desk of the supervisor who was the worst smoker, but it didn't help at all. Finally, the supervisor and another heavy smoker were moved into a side office. The other smokers in the office congregated there and the smoke was just as bad. It poured out into the hallways and other rooms.

Over the years, my asthma had gotten so much worse that I was taking maximum medication therapy, including steroids. I had chronic fatigue because I was unable to sleep more than a few hours a night between intermittent asthma attacks. It was difficult for me to function in any normal way because of my asthma. I couldn't walk a block outdoors, and I couldn't carry a sack of groceries without wheezing. The exertion of making a bed, sweeping a floor or doing laundry severely taxed my breathing. I could hardly find the strength after a day at the smoky office to stand in my kitchen and cook a meal. I had to eat standing up because sitting down while eating added strain to my already shallow breathing. It was hard for me to bend over to put shoes on, or to take a shower. I was just existing, trying to keep going so that we had my income. At work, I had to use my inhaler at closer and closer intervals to get through the workday; I had chronic laryngitis, found it hard to stand for long periods of time doing file work or to carry stacks of files down the hallway. My whole existence was simply to endure each working day and go home.

In October 1991, a new boss began harassing me. He confronted me at my desk in the reception room, right in front of other people sitting there, and said he didn't believe I was really ill. He forbade me to close the door or my office or the computer room in my effort to keep out smoke. He said there were "twenty-five of us and only one of you," and that the smokers had bent over backwards to accommodate me. He said I should look for another job. This time the union accepted the grievance I filed against him for harassing me and against the smoky conditions in the office.

My grievance went through three hearing levels and took three months. About half the office staff backed me, because they too wanted to see a smoke-free office. I had letters from coworkers past and present describing the awful smoke in the office. And of course I had copies of letters from my doctor to my supervisors and personnel office written over a period of the ten years. In December 1991, my office was designated completely nonsmoking.

But in October, two weeks after filing my grievance, my asthma was so bad I could no longer go on working. I could barely walk to my car after a day in the smoke. My medication was no longer helping me get through the days; I again filed for worker's compensation. I was away from work for three weeks. My doctor wanted me to return to work for as long as I could stand it in order to chart my breathing on a peak flow meter. As it turned out, my charting showed that I was then breathing half or less of my normal capacity, but it was a year before I was able to gauge my normal capacity. After returning to work for ten days, I was again too ill to continue, and left for another two weeks. During those absences or respites, I started being able to sleep a little, to walk around the house, and to breathe with less effort, enough to feel an improvement. I could not climb a flight of eight stairs to the shopping mall, stroll for half an hour in our local Japanese garden, or drive on vacation without being exhausted, but I started being able to sleep for a few hours without constant asthma attacks, and I could walk a few blocks slowly outdoors if it was a level surface.

In January 1992, after my office was designated nonsmoking, I returned to work. The rooms and hallways all smelled strongly of old smoke for many months afterward, and there were rooms that I couldn't walk past or enter without having an asthma attack from the lingering smell of smoke. My sense of smell improved the further away I got from the smoke at work. I still smelled fresh smoke coming through the air-conditioning vents in my office and in several other rooms. I realized it had to come from smokers in other parts of the building. (Other departments besides the district attorney's office occupied the courthouse.)

At the end of January, the county enacted an ordinance banning smoking in all county buildings, but the smoke kept coming through the ventilation system. I was still having occasional asthma attacks at work, although I was better away from the office. In March 1992, I contacted the building safety officer to discuss the smoke in the air-conditioning system of the building. The safety officer told me that no one had permission to smoke in the building, and he knew of no one who was smoking.

I filed my worker's comp case. I also filed a complaint against the county for discrimination and for failing to accommodate my health condition. The state department of air, employment, and housing prosecuted the case. I believe the attorneys who represented me did their best, but the outcome of that case in was discouraging. In a pretrial defense motion by the county, the judge dismissed my case because he said the county's nonsmoking ordinance enacted in 1992 was proof of accommodation of my disability. The judge heard no testimony about the lack of enforcement of the nonsmoking ordinance, or that smoke still existed in the air-conditioning system of the building that prevented me from working.

I don't know if I could have won with an expensive private attorney representing me, as happened with another person I know; she sued her private industry employer for assault and battery with smoke after she became ill with asthma while working in smoke for four years. She won her case in February 1994. It was also my bad luck to fall into the court of a judge who smoked and who previously worked for the district attorney's office; he took the county's ordinance at face value in making his ruling. The Department of Fair Employment decided not to re-file my case because it would have had to be heard again by the same judge. They decided not to file an appeal because they didn't have the manpower to continue working on it after nearly two years.

Over the next few months, I learned that public defenders, probation officers, a judge, and staff in the county clerk's office were smoking in their offices, in back hallways, in chambers and courtrooms, all in violation of the nonsmoking ordinance. I asked the safety officer to do something about it; he became evasive, claiming that no one was smoking. He said smoke could not reach the district attorney's office from other parts of the building, but suddenly was unable to locate the plans of the air-conditioning system to prove it. Other employees in my office and in the courtrooms also noticed smoke coming through the air conditioning and complained with me to the safety officer. Our complaints were fruitless. As the months progressed, my asthma, which had slightly improved early in the year with cessation of smoking in my immediate office, was again getting worse.

In July of 1992, I had a bad cold that lasted several weeks, during which time I completely lost my sense of smell. In late July, when I returned to work, the building's air conditioning malfunctioned for a week during a 100-degree heat wave. The day the air conditioning came back on I began having asthma attacks at my desk whenever gusts of air blew through the ventilation in the ceiling, even though I still could not smell. A coworker also started having allergic-type sneezing attacks and sinus infections. It wasn't until a week later that my sense of smell returned and I became aware of the smell of fresh burning tobacco smoke coming through the air conditioning. In October 1992, I was again unable to continue working and left on a worker's comp absence.

The emotional trauma of leaving my job in both 1991 and 1992 was devastating. I experienced depression, emotional numbness, periods of forgetfulness, constant weeping, anger, anxiety, hopelessness, and resignation. The psychiatrist who evaluated me for my worker's comp case apparently decided I had sustained no lasting emotional injury from this entire experience, so I did not qualify for any counseling. My only way to fight was by keeping records and writing letters. My doctor wrote a letter releasing me back to work in January 1993 with restrictions against any kind of smoke, and various chemicals that were common in the office: ammonia and other cleaning fluids, insecticide, and similar odorous items that were used around employees during office hours. My physical health continued to improve away from work. I still hoped to be able to return to my job. In March, I was notified I would not be accepted back at my job because of the chemical restrictions, but that I was welcome to seek an alternate assignment in the district attorney's office. Throughout the rest of 1993, I looked for a comparable job with nonsmoking conditions. Every office I checked for an alternate assignment had conditions similar to those where I worked, that is, people smoking stealthily in offices despite the complaints of others, or smoke circulating in the air conditioning from other offices in the building. In all my communications with my return-to-work coordinator in employee relations, the county refused to acknowledge, admit, or even address my concern that there was smoking in other county offices and buildings.

A year later, my worker's comp case was still pending. Because my employer contested it, I was not receiving any worker's comp benefits. I had been seen and examined by all the requisite physicians. The county refused to agree on a settlement. At the eleventh hour before each of several scheduled hearing dates, the county requested continuances. Then, they wanted me evaluated by yet two more independent doctors. I knew another woman, an asthmatic, who left her job with the county around the same time because of airborne irritants, and her worker's comp case has been pending for eight years.

When I left work in October 1992, I had worked for the county for twenty-four years. I was not eligible for retirement until fifty and after twenty-five years of service. To qualify for twenty-five years active service, I used all my accumulated vacation and sick time during my worker's comp absences. I still could not apply for retirement until my fiftieth birthday. The percentage of retirement benefits I could receive were minuscule compared to the wage I was earning, or to what I could have received in retirement benefits if I had been able to continue working another ten years. A year later my fifty-percent sick pay expired and I have been without funds since. I could not file for disability because my private physician, who had treated my asthma since 1983 and who advised me repeatedly not to return to work in the existing conditions, will not sign any more legal restrictions on my working and refused to help me file for disability. He thought I should just go find another job.

I still take medication to control my asthma and am vigilant about the environmental conditions to which I am exposed. My lungs are hypersensitive to the odor of smoke on the clothing of anyone near me or in a room with me. I cannot be in a house, motel room, office, shopping mall, or any other enclosed place where there is fresh or stale smoke in the air, air conditioning or clinging to carpeting or furnishing. Still, in the years I have been away from my job, my health has improved in a way I never would have expected.

It Is Difficult to Do This, to Bring Back All the Bad Memories, But Here Goes...—A Former Smoker

I've been exposed to secondhand smoke from the beginning; first, living with grandparents and smoking uncles, then through my mother's second marriage to a smoker, with friends who smoked, as well as my husband.

I began to smoke in my late teens when I started to work full-time. I think it was partly rebellion (mother disapproved) and social, as most of my friends and many fellow workers were smoking. I also had a boyfriend who smoked.

When I became pregnant with my first child at twenty-four, I found that smoking made me dizzy and sick. It was 1964 when the US Surgeon General began to make statements about the dangers of smoking. I think this may have been why I didn't resume smoking after the pregnancy—at least I like to think so.

My marriage ended after 15 years, I had been very ill with severe stomach problems and fatigue and was put on Tagamet, a common remedy for stomach conditions. I had been working for 12 years in a government office, with three years off for the birth of my second child. Here, again, I was constantly exposed to smoke from my fellow employees. I continued to work after the marital separation, as I had to support my children. My ex-husband was unable to help. The stomach problems and severe fatigue continued, and then, I began to have chest pains and soreness whenever I was near a cigar or pipe smoker. This caused much conflict with some fellow workers, and I also suffered immensely when I visited my mother and stepfather—he smoked a pipe. They live in Halifax, Nova Scotia, so when I visited them it meant I would be sleeping in their house. I needed the contact with my family, which included two half sisters and two half brothers. This is one of the worst psychological effects I suffered—being around people that I wanted to see made me suffer physical pain. One of my brothers and a brother-in-law also smoked, which further complicated matters. I have tried to encourage my son to persuade his wife not to smoke, as I'm concerned about him (he has allergies/bronchitis) and my grandchildren, as well as her. However, I don't push this much; it's too precarious being a "mother-in-law." She says she doesn't smoke around the children. I don't know how true this is, as they live in an apartment.

Eventually, all tobacco smoke began to affect me badly, as well as strong cleaning products, paint fumes, and to a lesser extent, perfumes. Thus began my horrible experience of trying to convince management at my workplace to provide me with an environment I could work in. This was 1986, and rumblings about smoke-free workplaces were beginning, but were meeting with much resistance. I talked to management, fellow workers, and union representatives. I tried being segregated from smokers, tried air purifiers, all with limited success. I had to keep working, as I was a single parent. I had to convince doctors to write letters on my behalf (not an easy task); my family physician was reluctant but finally gave in. I went to an allergist for skin tests; he found that I had many allergies, but when I didn't react to the skin prick for tobacco, he became hostile.

I was then off work for three months waiting to see a clinical ecologist (a specialist in environmental illness). He was very compassionate and helpful, and gave me many suggestions about nutrition, safe cleaning products, and other lifestyle changes I could implement to help myself. He also tested me for tobacco smoke sensitivity using a different method than skin pricks, and I reacted violently, shaking, coughing, heart racing, etc. We then decided I should try going back to work half-days, which I did. Meanwhile, there was a petition going around my workplace to see what people thought about going smoke-free. I certainly made a lot of enemies, but also had many on my side. I was working in a three-story building with about two hundred and fifty employees. I had also filed a grievance through my union and instructed my personnel office that I wished to apply for workers' compensation. The grievance was denied after many months. The personnel officer told me the workers' compensation application had been forwarded, but this turned out to be a lie. When I later contacted workers' compensation to see how things were progressing, they had no record of my complaint. After confronting personnel, the application was sent, but it was also eventually denied. I continued working half-days, when smoking was banned in all our offices. I was gradually able to go back to working full-time.

During all this time, my social life was very limited. Spontaneity went out the window. Any invitation to friends' or relatives' homes had to be refused if there would be any smokers there. Sometimes smokers would refrain or go outside if weather permitted, but there was always tension and embarrassment, and often hostility. I was a member of parents without partners for several years. The only activities I attended were theater outings and the occasional outdoor event. Restaurants were a problem, as well as dances and weddings. They still are. I lost some friends and had to give up seeing very much of my closest (geographically) relatives (an uncle and his wife who live near Toronto). However, I did adapt to this period of social isolation and was pleased when smoking became more and more socially unacceptable. I did quite well for a few years, changing my lifestyle completely to one of eating nutritious foods, avoiding foods identified as allergens, and trying to avoid chemicals and perfume as much as possible.

Unfortunately, in early 1990 I had difficulties again at work due to air-conditioning problems and continual renovations. I recovered from that after a while by working part-time again. Then again, in 1992, I became sick because of additional building renovations. I was working part-time again, and finally, I was having so many problems I applied for disability benefits and/or medical retirement—I now have full-blown environmental illness. Perfumes are now almost as big a problem as cigarette smoke, and harder to avoid. I was denied disability, but my medical retirement was approved so I now live on less than half of my full salary: a severe financial hardship.

I would say that the worst psychological effect of this forced life of semi-isolation is the loss of self-esteem because I feel that I can't "keep up with the pack." There is much depression, despair and loneliness, cynicism, and rage. I envy healthy people, or even those with other illnesses who are able to be with other people without adding to their pain. I also must deal with fear and anxiety whenever I have to go anywhere, always wondering whether I'll run into smokers, perfume wearers, etc. I've become very cynical, and there has been a definite loss of resilience in bouncing back from the emotional upsets of life. As I've become sicker, I've become less and less tolerant of smokers and their whining about addiction. At least it is possible to beat an addiction; if it is difficult to quit, it is not impossible. However, I'm left with an irreversible illness not of my own doing, and therein lies the difference. I'm also much more limited than most smokers are, which makes me furious!

To end on a positive note, for all the lost friends, I've made others like myself. I've also become a committed environmentalist in all aspects; I am very concerned about all pollution, indoor and outdoor, and make my views about the dangers of smoking, using pesticides, perfumes, etc., known whenever possible. I try not to preach and recognize when to shut up, even if it's difficult and I probably don't always succeed. However, that's one nice thing about getting older; one doesn't worry so much about what others think.

Since I'm now not working, I've taken on the presidency of a local allergy and environmental health group, which keeps me somewhat occupied and in touch with others with similar situations. It's a self-help group. It gives me some sense of accomplishment and the ability to share what I've learned with others. I also do a fair bit of phone counseling with people who sometimes just need to talk and get things off their chest.

Although I've been close to suicide a couple times, I'm still here and finding some pleasure in life. I do have some resourcefulness left, I guess, and a good sense of irony and sarcasm. I'll often force myself to watch comics on TV if I'm very depressed, or go to the library or joke books, as laughter really is the best medicine, as the saying goes. To quote a local doctor much sought after on the subject of healing with humor, "Laughter will inoculate you against the grumps, and you'll have fewer scowl movements in your life."

At the Age of Nine I Was Addicted—A Former Smoker

I grew up in a family of smokers. I was the youngest of three kids. My brother is ten years older, and my sister seven years older—both of them smoke still. I was raised on an Air Force base in a typical dysfunctional family. The first time I ever smoked a cigarette, I was seven years old. My parents used to have a rolling machine, so it was easy to steal cigarettes. When my mother caught me, I would receive some mild form of punishment. In those days, in the sixties, not much was publicized about the ill effects of smoking. I continued to smoke without inhaling until I was about nine. By then I was addicted, and when I was thirteen my mother had given up punishing me—my parents decided I could smoke at home.

My parents fought a lot. I was left to do pretty much what I wanted to do growing up. They could not control me. It was not long into my thirteenth year that I began to experiment with other drugs. I believe that when there is neglect at home a child searches for other forms of attention. I would try to get attention anyway I could from anyone who would give it.

There is a lot of power in being a child smoker. I felt strong and tough; I felt I could handle anything the world dished out to me. This feeling of invincibility led me to other drugs. I followed the typical path of a lot of young people. At sixteen, I was pregnant. I had quit doing drugs but not smoking cigarettes. I continued to smoke until 1981, when I quit for the first time. My boyfriend, Bill, now my husband, had never smoked, and cigarettes repulsed him. On a dare, I quit smoking. For the first week, I was unable to control my emotions and cried every time someone looked at me. The next three weeks were hard, but I managed not to smoke. At the time, I did not want to quit; I had only quit for Bill. I often thought about smoking and told myself that I would smoke again the minute Bill and I broke up.

Four years later, we did break up; I started smoking again. Bill and I got back together six months later, I didn't tell him I was smoking again. Keeping it secret was very stressful—I would try and find every excuse I could think of to go and have a cigarette.

It was not long after we got back together that I became pregnant with my second child. I then quit smoking again, this time for the baby. It was about six months after my son was born that I began smoking again. Bill and I married about a year later. It was sometime after our wedding that Bill found out my smoking secret. It was quite a shock for him; he had no idea I was smoking. It caused some friction in our marriage, but I never smoked in front of him or the kids. I became pregnant again two years later and quit again. Again, after my daughter was born I started smoking. Bill was constantly harassing me, and I demanded he lay off. I felt I was an adult and it was my choice to smoke; it was also my choice when to quit. Instead of trying to find excuses to go and have a cigarette, I could now smoke outside my house, and in the winter, the basement. I still did not smoke in front of my husband or children.

I always felt I wanted to quit and knew there were psychological reasons for my smoking. I knew the addiction was strong, but I had quit three times before and the last two times were not too difficult—there were no effects at all. When I delved deeper, I discovered that I smoked because of a lack of self-esteem. I am ambitious, and my pursuits were in the entertainment business as a musician/singer/songwriter. I made a lot of sacrifices for my marriage and children—things don't always go the way you hope. I had built up a lot of resentment and discovered that smoking was the one thing that no one could take away from me. I knew there was probably more to my smoking, but I was unable to reach deep enough to quit. I wanted to quit, but I couldn't…yet.

Five years after the birth of my last daughter, we moved to San Francisco to pursue our musical careers. We had done all we could in Canada and were finding it economically stagnant. It was about six months after we moved that I started to feel that I had sacrificed a great amount in the name of love. Now I felt that I had allowed the situation to get out of hand; I needed to take control of my life. I decided that I needed to make some changes—they would be slow, but I knew they would also lead to my quitting smoking.

For a singer, smoking is not a good thing. I would constantly ask myself, "If singing is so important to you why do you jeopardize it with cigarettes?" Bill and I did some goal-setting exercises, and I put a date to my next time to quit. I knew the next time I would quit it would be for me. Bill realized that and never pressured me further. My proposed quitting date was July 1, 1993.

On May 1, 1993, I smoked my last cigarette. It wasn't planned. I was sitting outside my house where I always smoked. It was the last cigarette in my package and I had two choices at that moment: quit or buy another pack. I walked into the house and told Bill I had quit smoking. Of course, he didn't really think I was serious. Not much was said about it, but I have not smoked since.

What happened to me after quitting this time was very different than any other time. Everything seemed to be going well. Naturally, I had cravings and sometimes felt like giving in, but about a month after I quit I went into complete mental breakdown. I was at work and feeling hostile, then I became very emotional. My boss was alerted and came to see me. He knew I had quit smoking and asked if that was the problem. I denied it emphatically; I told him it was the pressures of life. I was angry that anyone would think I could be depressed and lost just because of smoking.

It was about three months after that I realized it was the smoking that had caused so much of my anxiety. It was as if the world had opened up and I was standing in the middle and everyone was looking in at me. I felt my whole soul was exposed. Most people I tell this to think I'm a little strange. I felt my whole life had been affected by smoking, every decision, every choice, and every excuse I made to not go forward with my life. I have always prided myself on the fact that I was in control of my senses. I had quit doing drugs when I was sixteen because I didn't like being out of control. All of a sudden, I realized that every decision I had made in the past was actually related to smoking.

I would try to practice my guitar, but that would only last until I craved a cigarette. We have a recording studio in our home, and if Bill needed me to sing it was always a problem because I wasn't able to smoke; it caused unnecessary friction when we worked together. Because I didn't smoke in front of my family, if I had to go on an errand and my kids wanted to come along, I would say no—I sacrificed time with my children so I could smoke a cigarette! I was thinking about quitting my part-time job, but before I could do it I would weigh if I would be able to smoke so freely at my next job. When our nonsmoking friends invited us out, I had to plan out where I could have a cigarette before I said yes, and if it meant I could only have one cigarette before I got back home, I said I decided I didn't feel like going out. Every move, every day, every moment, every thought was planned around having a cigarette.

When I discovered that cigarettes controlled my whole life, I broke down. It was extremely frightening to me to realize that they had such control over me. I imagine it to be like an awakening with multiple personalities meeting each other for the first time. When I became aware of what had happened I cried for all the experiences I missed with my family, friends, and career. I had jeopardized a lot in the name of a cigarette.

Back to the present: I just celebrated an anniversary as a nonsmoker. I am not a born-again nonsmoker. I do not preach about the ill effects or the psychological effects of smoking to other smokers. I was a smoker; I know the anxieties of the addiction, as with any other addiction, you cannot convince a smoker of what they are doing to themselves. It is an internal struggle that can only be won within oneself.

I still have the occasional craving and probably always will. When I first quit smoking, I used to be envious of the people I saw who could drink and smoke all day long. Thankfully, those thoughts went away and I am getting my life in order.

CHAPTER 8

Why Smoke?

People begin to smoke and continue the habit for numerous reasons. While most recall smoking their first cigarette as a young person, especially in adolescence, some do pick up the habit much later in life. Of those who begin as youth and young adults, many makers resent growing up around role models who smoked, including parents and other close relatives, teachers, coaches, heads of churches, movie stars, as well as peers. These youth choose to smoke in imitation of role models because they simply want to be like the adults or peers they admire and to feel "grown up," to "fit in," to "be cool" or "one of the guys."

Some believe that the desire to fit in that leads them to smoke is directly related to low self-esteem; smoking made them feel important and adult. Additionally, to smoke is to be rebellious—the teenager's raison d'être. And, like many consumers, young adults often believe the advertising: smoking embodies sophistication, glamor, and mystery. Access is essential to becoming a smoker, and smokers who start smoking particularly early in their lives generally have parents who smoke or close friends whose parents smoke. Young adults also pick up the habit from coworkers who smoke, and college students are as likely to pick up the habit from their peers as their younger counterparts. Finally, many young men started smoking in military service because of access to free or cheap cigarettes.

Those who pick up the habit later in life also do so for a variety of reasons: some report smoking to control their weight, to emulate another who smokes, and even to self-medicate on the advice of other smokers.

I. Newman and J. DeFrain, *Tobacco Use and Intimate Relationships*,
https://doi.org/10.1007/978-3-319-92579-0_8

Many smokers hold to the belief that smoking is a cure for various ailments, particularly stress and anxiety. One woman, for example, started smoking for a sore throat; her husband recommended menthol cigarettes. Unfortunately, many smokers have refused to quit or resumed smoking after quitting for a time because they fear weight gain. For many respondents who smoke, obesity is seemingly worse than tobacco addiction. Interestingly, both smokers and the obese are visible populations generally rejected by mainstream society. Smokers, like the obese, are considered weak-willed/minded people with no self-control or sense of self-preservation. Consequently, perceived as un-adult for their "unhealthy habits," they are often vulnerable to public abuse and treated patronizingly.

Why smokers continue to light up and inhale is much simpler: addiction, stressful lives, and pure pleasure. Cigarettes quickly become integral to one's daily routine, and the smoker soon cannot imagine getting through the day without the repeated ritual of lighting up, holding onto and inhaling the smoke of a cigarette. For these smokers, cigarettes are like a close companion and friend, present through all the trials of life and therefore difficult, sometimes impossible, to let go. Others wax poetic about the sensuality of smoking and love everything about the cigarette—its smell, the smoke, and the physical ritual of smoking.

The time and place in which one lives is also crucial to whether or not people begin to smoke and the lifespan of their smoking habit. Many older smokers began smoking in the fifties, when the habit was socially acceptable (even recommended), and everyone seemed to smoke. Even though the Surgeon General's warning about tobacco use came out in the sixties, open acknowledgment of the dangers of tobacco use, smoking regulations, and the anti-smoking sentiments of today are still fairly recent.

Where one lives—for example, California versus North Carolina—can also determine whether one begins or continues to smoke.

Testimony

For the past twenty years I have been waking every hour throughout the night for a cigarette. I smoke twenty-four hours a day and ***there is not one cigarette that I do not enjoy or look forward to.*** *(a smoker who can't quit)*

*****

As unbelievable as it is to me now, by the time I was fifteen I too was hooked by the secondhand smoke where I hung out as a teenager. That coupled with ***my desire "to be a man" and fit in and be "cool"; I decorated my room with Marlboro ads and cigarette flip-top boxes!*** *It wasn't until I turned twenty-three that I was able to hear how horrible smoking was, with the help of a relentless roommate who was sickened by my habit, and I finally quit. (a former smoker)*

*****

My husband, Don, was very gentle. ***Sometimes I think he needed smoking to bolster his ego****. (a lifelong nonsmoker)*

*****

*...peer pressure helped—****everyone I knew smoked Marlboros.*** *(a smoker who can't quit)*

*****

I tried smoking three times. Dad would throw his lit cigarettes off the porch—I picked one up once while playing on the lawn and took a puff. I was about ten at the time. Later, five of us girls who ran around together went to one girl's house on lunch break. She lived a block from our high school. We all tried a couple of cigarettes. I was fifteen. Then in my late thirties I thought I'd try smoking to lose weight. I tried it a couple of times and hated it. (a lifelong nonsmoker)

*****

My childhood peers considered me a nerd. I lived in a fairly isolated residential cluster set amidst a small farming community fifteen miles from town. About the only social interaction available was with a neighborhood gang comprised of around twenty-five youths my age and older. All of these kids were smokers, and a large part of my early smoking was to gain peer-group acceptance. Also, ***my father, grandfather, my uncle (who lived with us) all smoked, as did my physician, teacher, Episcopal priest, bishop and local politicians. My president, F.D.R., was seldom seen without his famous cigarette holder.*** *Tobacco advertising was rampant, "Camels—not a cough in a carload." And, "More doctors have switched to Camels than any other* *brand." Also, "Lucky Strike green has gone to war," alluding to the green printer's ink that went into the package. (a former smoker)*

*****

I smoke now. ***I wanted to be like my mom, so I started when I was ten.*** *(a smoker who can't quit)*

*****

When I was twenty-one years old in college, one of my roommates gave me a cigarette because I was stressed over exams and term papers. When I finally finished school and got my first job in a laboratory, I continued to smoke because it was hectic with hardly any time for breaks. Smoking helped. The only time I would stop and rest was when I had a cigarette, so I believed that it was relaxing. ***I enjoyed smoking. It is hard for nonsmokers to understand this, but it's true.*** *(a former smoker)*

*****

I began to smoke in my late teens when I started to work full-time. I think it was partly rebellion (mother disapproved) and social, *as most of my friends and many fellow workers were smoking. I also had a boyfriend who smoked. (a former smoker)*

*****

I took up smoking because I felt it helped my anxiety and loneliness. *(a former smoker)*

*****

I started smoking at thirteen, mainly because everyone else did it and I wanted to be cool. *Almost all my friends smoked, and it didn't take long for me to get hooked. (a former smoker)*

*****

I think one of the things that got me started was how my peers and current movie stars glamorized smoking. ***They all smoked, and of course they all made a big thing about how they lit their cigarettes. People like John***

Wayne, Humphrey Bogart and Charlie Chan made it look glamorous. *Anyway, it wasn't long before I was addicted to tobacco. (a former smoker)*

*****

Cigarettes are nasty; they stink up everything and the ashes are filthy. Cigarettes make smoker's breath just awful, and even the house furnishings and walls get tinted gray with cigarette smoke. I can't understand why anyone would want to put these things into their bodies; people never seem to learn. Even if one has a parent who smokes and sees the damage done, they still smoke. My oldest sister smokes today and she has definitely seen the results. All of this doesn't even touch the amount of money a person burns each time they light up. I have no idea what they cost, but years ago when my mother smoked the price of cigarettes was outrageous. (a former smoker)

*****

When I was about eight or nine we had rabbit tobacco growing in a field next to our house. Once, when my aunt was visiting from St. Louis, she pointed it out and showed us how they used to smoke it rolled up in pieces of brown paper bag. My siblings and I tried smoking it and would smoke it whenever it was in season. ***Though my mom and dad were opposed to us smoking, for some reason they thought it was cute that we smoked the rabbit tobacco, and they overlooked it.*** *I began smoking seriously about the time I got to junior high when smoking in general and in the boys' room was considered cool—Rebellion, I suppose. I knew that my parents did not want me to smoke.* ***Peer pressure played a huge part in it as all the guys I hung around with smoked; it was a sign of nonconformity to the powers that be at school and at home. My brother and sister and I got more than one whipping because we were caught smoking.*** *(a smoker who can't quit)*

*****

I tried smoking when I was about fifteen, but I didn't continue. Then, when I was about seventeen, ***I thought cigarettes would calm my nerves and give me something to do. You might say I did it out of boredom—no one ever pressured me to smoke. I enjoyed my new "hobby." I thought it was fun to buy cigarettes. I felt like I was part of a group, accepted by other smokers. It was like having "friends." I enjoyed puffing away after a cup of coffee or a meal; it soothed me. I felt important when I smoked.*** *(a former smoker)*

*****

I quit smoking for six months after I had back surgery and then I picked up the habit again after gaining too much weight. *I worked out for 5 days a week and could not lose the weight. (a smoker who can't quit)*

*****

I started smoking as a high school teen because of peer pressure. I was fourteen or fifteen years old. All my friends did if and all the girls I went out with smoked. ***It was the thing to do. I continued to smoke because I really liked it.*** *(a smoker who can't quit)*

*****

My first experience with smoking was at an early experimental stage with my brother and friends. ***All our parents smoked. Cigarettes were always readily available in fancy cigarette boxes around the house. We would smoke to look, act, and play like grown-ups. We were raised with cigarette advertising all around us—the Marlboro Man, "You've Come a Long Way Baby," and others.*** *Women were sophisticated, elegant and "sexy" if they smoked. I began smoking seriously at sixteen. I had moved to Long Island from a small town in southern New Jersey and was very lonely. I had also put on a great deal of weight and was miserable. I made friends with peers who smoked, and after my many days of "trying" cigarettes at a younger age, I knew how to do it well—it was easy. My mother allowed me to smoke in the house because she knew I would anyway. She bought me cigarettes and I purchased them myself at local stores; getting cigarettes was never a problem. (a smoker who can't quit)*

*****

It was a powerful habit that I tried to break many, many times, especially when suffering a bout of pleurisy or bronchitis. Even before all the hoopla about the bad effects, I was very much aware that it was doing me irrevocable harm. ***"They" say that smokers have low self-esteem—I think this is a problem that stems from not being in control of one's life enough to be able to quit. That is at least true in my case.*** *(a former smoker)*

*****

…tobacco was like new-mown hay. ***The taste, the fragrance and the aroma were a sensual pleasure.*** *I shared the enjoyment of tobacco with my best friends. The pleasures of tobacco include fun, pleasure, taste and convenience:*

the aroma, the taste satisfaction without the guilt of fattening calories. Also, my hay fever and sinus allergies, frequently a cause of agony and suffering, subsided with smoking. (a former smoker)

*****

Although I hated my first cigarette, I continued to smoke until I was hooked. ***At first, I liked the feel of the cigarette between my fingers. I liked the way the smoke curled when I exhaled, and after a meal, a cigarette "tasted good," although now I cannot imagine ever thinking that. But most of all, everyone else smoked.*** *(a former smoker)*

*****

I don't know why I began smoking so late in life. I never imagined I would ever smoke and don't know exactly why I began. I had no role models, but a lover of mine used to speak wistfully of his ex-wife and her smoking as an "enigma"; she became someone I envied. *So, I taught myself to smoke. It was terrible at first and I tried it many times, trying different brand each day. I practiced being cool and mysterious until one day, about a week later, the menthol started tasting good to me. I wanted to look better and it tasted good for a few years. My awareness of myself as an individual increased. I began to assert my decision to smoke even if sometimes others did not like it. An added bonus was that my hay fever and allergies subsided—RELIEF! (a former smoker)*

*****

I started smoking at sixteen in high school; I wanted to be a "regular guy" and smoke like all the other "guys." Father was a smoker and wouldn't allow me to smoke until I was sixteen. ***At first I smoked to feel "big." It was WWII that set it in concrete; I was in heavy combat, so when I was able to rest and smoke it was the world's greatest comfort, next to still being alive. Today it's the taste, mildness, menthol and cost that attract me to smoke.*** *(a smoker who can't quit)*

*****

I began smoking at thirteen. For years I wondered how I ever began; the practice is so repugnant to me. Looking back, I think it was a "rite of passage." I really hated the smell, look and taste of tobacco; yet, like a mindless body I was attracted to it. Both my mother and grandmother smoked. ***I remember feeling real "cool." I practiced the coolest way of smoking, holding the cigarette and blowing smoke rings. It made me feel glamorous.*** *I smoked for years. I never tried to quit—I never even thought about it. I worked in public places like restaurants, lounges and clubs; I did not know any nonsmokers. (a former smoker)*

*****

I started smoking on a regular basis after I entered the military. It was what "real men" did. (a former smoker)

*****

My eighteen-year history with nicotine began in 1973 at the age of fourteen. I remember that in 1973 not much was known about the harms of smoking cigarettes. ***Smoking was publicized as glamorous or cool. My circle of friends and I were typical, mildly rebellious teenagers. All of us had at least one parent who smoked. We stole cigarettes from our parents and dared each other to smoke them. When we started buying cigarettes at the local stores, no sales clerks ever refused to sell them to us.*** *It would take us weeks to finish one pack. We continued at this pace until high school. (a former smoker)*

*****

My husband bought me a pack of Salems and said the menthol would help my throat and sinuses and make me feel better, so I tried them. *At first I choked and felt dizzy, but they did help me feel better. Maybe it was relaxing me or maybe the menthol helped, although another form of menthol like Vicks would have been safer. After that I smoked two or three cigarettes a day, sometimes more. Sometimes I smoked my husband's unfiltered Camels. They were awful. After about eight years I gradually went up to three-fourths of a pack a day. My husband smoked a pack and a half daily. After about ten years, Salem changed so I started smoking Kool, then Kool Lights 100s. (a smoker who can't quit)*

*****

My husband and I started smoking in our teens—he at sixteen, me at eighteen. I started because he smoked; he started because his friends smoked. *We are now seventy-one and sixty-seven. He smoked regularly for fifty years; I smoked for forty-five years. The addiction is frightful. As anyone who* *has been a smoker knows, the habit builds and builds. I started with two or three cigarettes a day; when I finally quit four years ago, I was smoking over one-and-a-half packs per day. (a former smoker)*

*****

It was the thing to do. I bought cigarettes in every color to match my outfits. Can't you see me now? Sixteen years old, a size eight, straw hat, white gloves, suit, heels, hose and cigarettes to match: "Ain't she sweet?" *(a smoker who can't quit)*

*****

Both my single parent-family status and an IQ above the ninety-ninth percentile set me apart from my peer group. I eagerly sought acceptance, but that was difficult to attain. In fact, until I reached full maturity ***I strove for peer acceptance in every way that I could in a futile attempt to appear "normal." I'm quite certain, at least in retrospect, that this was the underlying motivation for me to begin smoking at such an early and impressionable age and later to continue smoking.*** *I took up smoking to "be one of the guys," enlisted in the navy and volunteered for submarine duty. (a former smoker)*

*****

Every role model that I can recall was a smoker. My mother remarried when I was twelve, and both my stepfather and his father—whom I particularly admired—were smokers. My parish priest and the bishop of our Episcopal Diocese smoked, as well as my physician, local politicians and community leaders, General Douglas McArthur, President Franklin Delano Roosevelt, and my hero, John Wayne. One of my high school sports coaches was a chain-smoker, and I recall even now the very obvious yellow stains on his fingers attesting to his cigarette habit. (a former smoker)

Stories

It's Been a Source of Very Angry Disagreements Between Us—A Former Smoker

When I was growing up in the fifties, my parents were both heavy smokers. As kids, my two brothers and I complained a lot about them smoking in the car. They would simply tell us to "crack the window a bit." As they were very considerate, respectable and well-liked people, it seemed a little strange that they wouldn't refrain from smoking in the car.

My mother was a meticulous housekeeper and would always despair as she scrubbed at the terrible brown residue on walls, ceilings, and woodwork from smoking. She washed the curtains, aired drapes, bedding, and clothing in a regular cycle of spring and fall housecleaning, and frequently in between, often declaring the need to air things out. So while I received the impression that cigarette smoke was dirty and smelly, I never felt it was dangerous, that is, until my baby brother was born small and premature when I was twelve. The doctor told my mother that the reason for his low birth weight was that she smoked during her pregnancy. She disputed that because I had been an eight-pound baby and she smoked before I was born, as with my middle brother.

Smoking was frequently cited as a way of calming my mother's nerves, and she always grabbed her cigarettes when the phone rang. She's seventy-six and still does this.

When I was at high school only the wild girls at our Catholic school smoked, but once I was in teachers college a friend I was rooming with convinced me to at least try it. I have a photograph of myself practicing in front of a mirror. I felt very mature. At school, we were required to go into the furnace room to smoke, but since most of the staff was in there, except the nuns, it was decided to build a staff room when an addition was put on the school. The students joked about the billows of smoke emerging from the staff room windows at recess and lunch hour.

All the young men I dated smoked, and although I did not enjoy it, I felt a need to be part of the group. I usually only smoked when someone else was present, chose menthol brands, avoided inhaling, and religiously washed my hair and aired my clothes after major smoke-filled gatherings.

Each time I lit up my eyes watered and my nose ran; often I would sneeze several times during the first few puffs. Everyone thought it was hilarious that I continued to smoke, but I remember insisting that I enjoyed it. Though untrue, I thought it necessary to avoid being labeled uptight. The few times I smoked marijuana I hated the acrid smoke but loved being "with-it" even more.

I quit smoking during my first pregnancy and gave birth to a premature, low-weight baby who suffered brain damage because of oxygen deprivation. This caused me such stress I began to smoke again when he was just a few months old. I smoked during my second pregnancy and had a healthy seven-pound boy. I even smoked while I was nursing him. When the kids were little my husband and I both quit several times. I attempted to quit once after one child was accidentally burned on the finger, and another time after I found one holding a cigarette lighter.

In the eighties, I returned to teaching, but only smoked during breaks at school and on weekend social gatherings. Both of my sons experimented with cigarettes between the ages of twelve and fifteen. One of them resumed smoking at college and the other never pursued it after the first few tries. He has epilepsy as a result of birth trauma and takes massive doses of medication to control his seizures.

The psychological addiction is almost greater than the physical one. It's so hard to break the habit of having coffee with a cigarette, chatting on the phone and smoking, especially when others around you are.

When I was in my early forties, smoking more and enjoying it less, I came to grips with the stupidity of it all. I finally quit cold turkey in total disgust and became a strong anti-smoking lobbyist despite the fact that my husband continued to smoke a pack a day. It has been a source of many angry disagreements between us and the cause of much sadness. I've tried to rationalize his addiction as more powerful than his concern for me, but it doesn't always help. He smokes in the house, especially during the winter, and I complain a lot about the smell and brown deposit it leaves. When he lost his job three years ago, I begged him to quit; cigarettes were very expensive. He insists on buying only a pack at a time. I got him a prescription for patches—he never used them. Nor did he use the gift certificate for hypnosis I gave him. We continue to argue daily about smoking. My husband is a very loving, kind, helpful man, but this issue is putting a serious strain on our twenty-eight-year marriage life.

My mother recognizes my sensitivity to cigarette smoke but continues to smoke in my presence. I have made it known to guests in my home that I prefer that they smoke outside, weather permitting, or in the basement. My mother disregards this request. I have always asked her not to smoke around her grandchildren but she still does at her house, although not at theirs. She continues to offer my son and his girlfriend cigarettes when we are all together, but she asks them not to smoke near me.

A few years ago my mother was constantly clearing her throat and complaining about difficulty swallowing. It turned out that she had throat polyps and had to have surgery to remove them. Four days later she started smoking again. At seventy-six she says she's not quitting because you have to die of something. We often discuss smoking. She did quit for a few months but is back at it again.

Smoking is an addiction of serious proportions and not recognized as the health issue it really is. If we have seat belt laws and anti-littering laws, it's hard to believe that enforcing a no-smoking ban is impossible on this continent!

To Be the "Inspiration" to Your Kids to Smoke Is a Rotten Legacy to Leave with Your Children—A Former Smoker

I was about twenty years old when it became "cool" to smoke. I learned to smoke, and the addiction stayed with me until I was sixty-six—a long time to be stupid! I started about a year before college, but not in a serious, frequent way. Smoking was easy then. The majority of my friends and associates were smokers: nurses, our family physician, my college roommate, my girlfriend, other students, professors; everyone smoked. One of my favorite teachers said he smoked to "toughen his throat against colds and infections." He died of lung cancer.

Smoking was enjoyable. The advertisements buttressed these "benefits." In the Army, the tobacco companies were always giving their products away. Wartime commercials always told of their carloads of gifts to the armed forces. If the enemy didn't get us, the tobacco companies would.

It was accepted and relatively inexpensive. As far as I can recall, there was no substantial outcry or warning from the medical industry, which to many minds, including mine, meant that except for a few minor negatives like fire hazards, the stink and dirty ashes, smoking was an acceptable and okay practice. After all, our actors, actresses, and sports heroes were doing it, and the Chesterfield slogan, "They satisfy," kind of said it all. We needed that kind of support for our foolishness.

Like many smokers I knew, or know, I quit smoking many times. Intuition and, later, more and more opposition from the medical community and other health organizations were beginning to raise doubts about the "benefits" of smoking. The tide was beginning to turn—granted, late, but the tobacco industry and its allies were beginning to lose!

I quit smoking dozens of times; there was nothing to it! But dozens of times I went back to the weed. I knew I was addicted when I was in the Army. We were bottled up in forward positions and would run out of cigarettes for five or six days. I'd thought about quitting; there would be just one less thing to lug around. At the end of a siege, instead of using those five or six days as a jump on quitting the "habit," I lit up again as soon as cigarettes were sent to us—Hooked again!

I will always deeply regret having smoked. We have six children, four of whom smoked. Three still smoke (one is now trying to quit). To have "inspired" your kids to smoke is a rotten legacy.

Talking to our children was not forceful enough, and in most cases, we were ignored. I feel that it's way late now, but hopefully not too late to be more vocal and open about my opposition. However, I find it difficult to admonish our children and even a grandchild who we caught smoking at thirteen—A twinge of hypocrisy hits me, I guess. I tried singing a song I heard some twenty-five to thirty years ago to my grandchild: "Puff, puff that cigarette…Puff, puff it till you're almost dead" (or words to that effect). The finale was a true analysis of the smoker: "…a fire on one end and a fool on the other." The reaction to my singing was a look that said, "There he goes again."

I failed this time, but I will keep trying. The old guilt and hypocrisy thing kept me quiet. But now my view is changing. I think our thirteen-year-old grandchild blew my objections away, but that's a poor excuse for silence. Another side effect of tobacco addiction is stealth. Like others I knew who tried to quit, I found myself becoming sneaky. We became closet dwellers, an introduction to a negative lifestyle.

Some years ago a doctor friend who was an ex-smoker advised me to quit, telling me that cold turkey was the only way to go, although "it ain't easy." Making up my mind to do it was difficult; actually quitting was not half as bad as I expected. Others supported my efforts, but did not consider it very important.

I Would Do Anything to Get One—A Former Smoker

I was an eighteen-year-old college freshman experimenting with cigarettes with other girls on my dorm floor. Several had smoked for a while. No one in my immediate family smoked. I had a boyfriend at the time who smoked a pipe and came from a family of smokers.

I initially started smoking because I thought it was a "grown-up" thing to do; I was surrounded by college friends who smoked, and I wanted to try it. I remember sitting in a dorm room one Friday night trying to learn to inhale. I just couldn't get the hang of it. I smoked for a month before I learned to inhale. I thought I looked mature smoking, and probably did it because I was trying out my newfound freedom—being away from home.

I liked it. I've always liked the taste, the feeling of relaxation that I felt as I smoked, and at one time I even liked the smell of tobacco. I kept my smoking "secret" from my parents for ten to twelve years, and in more than twenty years of smoking, I never smoked around them. I only smoked cigarettes around my sister. I could go without cigarettes for long periods of time as long as I knew I'd eventually be able to have one. For several years I smoked a half to one pack a day, never more.

I really enjoyed smoking—I found it relieved my uptight nature. Smoking calmed me. I always have things in my mouth like pens, pencils. I think my smoking at first was an oral gratification thing. However, I soon found it was an addiction, not so much caused by the need for tobacco but a habit. I found I could go without smoking for two weeks when I went on trips with my family and never crave a cigarette or really even think about it. But as soon as I got back home, I'd run out and buy cigarettes.

I found I didn't like sneaking around, but even in later years, I lied about my smoking. When I married, I promised my husband that I would quit smoking. He disapproved of smoking. However, I never did quit. When we divorced, he was the one who spilled the beans and told my family I smoked. I knew my parents would disapprove if they ever found out, especially since my mother was a nurse and had warned me of the side effects of smoking.

My friends over the years were all smokers. During my twenties and thirties, the smoking group always seemed to be the group I fit in with and enjoyed. Cigarettes were common ground for us. We'd meet at parties and it always seemed that cigarettes were the reason we got along. We all seemed to be the same type of individuals.

For the past two to three years I have tried to quit—I switched to lower tar and nicotine brands and reduced the number of cigarettes I smoked daily. I got down to one cigarette a day for six months then I started up again, but for two years I kept my intake to less than ten a day. I wanted to quit only because I knew it was bad for my health; I suffered from bronchitis frequently.

The most difficult part for me was to tell myself I had to quit because I truly enjoyed it, even now wish I were still smoking. I miss it: the taste, the action, and the relaxation. I have to constantly tell myself that it's for my own good that I not smoke.

My friends (who all smoke) encouraged me when I first quit and were supportive. I am the first one in my group to quit.

I knew I was addicted to tobacco when I tried to quit for the first time; I realized I wanted a cigarette in the worst way and would do anything to get one.

I still miss smoking and have had a hard time keeping from gaining weight, which was always my fear; I gained twenty pounds. I still have the desire for a cigarette and have even joked that if the doctor told me tomorrow that I only had a short time to live, I'd go back to smoking in a minute. I only quit because of all the information on the risks of cancer, but I can honestly say that I didn't want to quit. I know I won't slide now and start again, but I feel the desire will never leave me.

I'm a teacher/counselor and have told students to give it up while they can and before they become addicted.

CHAPTER 9

Quitting

Although quite a few smokers deny that they might be addicted to tobacco, claiming they can quit if they want to, most of the smokers in our study and many who have attempted to quit are quick to admit addiction. Many people only realize they are addicted when they attempt to quit—finding that it is no easy task. Quitting smoking (or even not being able to have one for an extended period) entails physical and mental anguish: Smokers face withdrawal symptoms, from nervousness to headaches, and constantly crave the release that can only come from a cigarette. Because quitting is so difficult, the process is usually a trial for everyone involved, particularly loved ones. Family members report the difficulties of dealing with a loved one attempting to quit and all the consequences of withdrawal.

The physical act of smoking—described as sensual by many—as much as the chemical effects of tobacco makes quitting very difficult for the majority of smokers. Cigarettes become an integral part of one's daily routine: morning coffee, after meals, talking on the telephone, driving, socializing with friends, evening cocktails, and times of stress as well as happiness. Lifestyle changes are necessary in order to reduce or quit smoking, something not very many of us have the discipline and will to enact. Furthermore, as many smokers fear weight gain, some who quit resume smoking after putting on weight. Clearly, lifestyle changes are necessary to quit and to remain smoke-free. Former smokers do not necessarily lose the desire to smoke. Former smokers who have quit years before admit to still wanting a cigarette occasionally, and some, believing

I. Newman and J. DeFrain, *Tobacco Use and Intimate Relationships*,
https://doi.org/10.1007/978-3-319-92579-0_9

themselves immune to addiction a second time, give into "one cigarette" only to relapse entirely. Some also give into the temptation of smoking during particularly stressful periods. Unfortunately, being successful at quitting the first time around does not guarantee success the next time, and some find that they cannot quit again.

Smokers attempt to quit for a variety of reasons. Those reasons can determine the success or failure of their efforts. For example, to quit because a loved one pressures you to quit often leads to secret smoking and resentment. Rarely are smokers able to quit unless they genuinely want to. Smokers who do want to quit are generally concerned about their health as well as the health of those around them. Unfortunately, many only quit for good when their health is in critical condition—after having been diagnosed with cancer and prior to radical treatment such as surgery.

The methods for quitting are numerous and costly: the patch, gum, stop-smoking programs, counseling, hypnosis, and acupuncture. Most former smokers report that the most successful method is going "cold turkey." Some smokers are able to do just that. Others must first reduce the number and frequency of cigarettes before quitting altogether.

Because it requires and entails lifestyle change, the process of quitting is an eye-opening experience for many smokers. Early in the process of attempting to quit, the realities of smoking as an addiction begin to set in, and the illusions of many that they are in control of the process inevitably fall to pieces. Such an experience can be traumatic and eventually freeing. While some former smokers still crave cigarettes, missing the sensations of smoking as well as its rituals, many learn to hate everything about smoking and cannot even image how they started in the first place. Some even become active in the anti-smoking movement—"born-again nonsmokers."

Testimony

Cigarettes consumed my days and nights; my first priority was to buy and smoke cigarettes. I have only quit for a year now, but cigarettes are still on my mind. Last week I took my first puff since I quit and coughed my lungs out. I don't miss it; ***those damned things have wasted so much of my life. I feel like I wasted twenty years.*** *(a former smoker)*

*****

Each time I quit I did it cold turkey without any help from anyone. I don't know if this is possible with drugs such as cocaine or heroin—it seems like most alcoholics have to have help and support to quit. So how do you define addiction? *I could also have become an alcoholic, but decided early in life that I would only drink socially. We have liquor in the house all the time. I suppose I have a drink every six months or so, maybe at Christmas or an anniversary. Addiction may well depend on one's will power. I can go for hours without a cigarette in situations where I can't smoke and still not lose my cool.* ***Am I an addict then; or do I smoke because I enjoy it?*** *(a smoker who can't quit)*

*****

I realize that I am addicted. ***Each time I quit I start up again, and the craving is always there.*** *(a smoker who can't quit)*

*****

So, even my two bouts with cancer have not stopped this terrible habit. It's pretty scary to know I have an addiction that has such a powerful hold on me. Also, I am worried about all the children and other people who do not deserve to be affected by our second-hand smoke. I feel we should be free to choose if we want to smoke or not, but I also feel that nonsmokers should not be subjected to our smoke invading their lungs and saturating their clothes. ***We smoke because we once chose to and now we smoke because we haven't the willpower to stop.*** *(a smoker who can't quit)*

*****

I am sure that I am addicted to nicotine. I don't know how I know except that I positively have to have a cigarette every few hours. *Only under the most dire circumstances can I go for more than two hours without a smoke. Most of the time I have a hard time going an hour without a cigarette unless I am real busy. I can stretch the time out by chewing gum, sucking candy or eating sunflower seeds, but I actually start trembling and feel weak if I have to go too long.* ***When I go without a smoke my mouth waters, the top of my mouth itches, I feel nervous and anxious and I get a headache. Is smoking pleasurable? Pleasurable can't be the right word. There is just nothing pleasurable about it; it is more like satisfying or gratifying the craving.*** *(a smoker who can't quit)*

*****

I am addicted. I may never quit—I don't know. ***When I try to quit I get down. I cry. I yell. I get critical.*** *I am normally a very happy, upbeat person. (a smoker who can't quit)*

*****

I am definitely addicted to tobacco. ***If I can't have a cigarette, all I do is think about it and want it more; it's the only thing on my mind. People who don't smoke don't understand. They think it's so easy to just not smoke when you crave a cigarette.*** *(a smoker who can't quit)*

*****

Yes, I am addicted. I like it very much and I don't want to quit. ***It's like ecstasy when I light up. If it is addiction, I am thoroughly enjoying it.*** *At least my tobacco is legal. (an unrepentant smoker)*

*****

I buy one pack a day. If I bought a carton I would smoke ten packs a week instead of seven. *I tried buying cigarettes that are on sale—cheap ones. They would hurt my lungs, so I went back to Carlton 100s each time: one milligram of nicotine and one milligram of tar. (a smoker who can't quit)*

*****

My addiction is such that about every fifty minutes or so I feel a strong urge to have one—throughout the day. *I usually go to bed at about ten and wake up at about four to go to the bathroom, and then I have to have a cigarette. If I'm with company I can usually hold out for a couple of hours. (a smoker who can't quit)*

*****

Three days ago I started wearing the patch to see if I could kick this rotten addiction. I put it on in the morning and I had to pull it off at about 6 p.m. because my heart felt like it would run away and the patch hurt. Usually I need to smoke one cigarette every morning around nine. Today I fought that desire. It is now close to noon and I'm still fighting. This is the first time I have felt like really fighting it for any length of time, and I can see that I'm in for a very rough time. ***My nerves are frazzled, my body is tense, and my mind befuddled. In my head I have a vision of cigarettes. I want one and it's all I can think about.*** *My body craves that cigarette and my mind must fight my body's desire. I pray and hope that I can make it. Even with a serious illness knocking at my door, this fight is extremely hard. (a smoker who can't quit)*

*****

I have enjoyed smoking for many years and have never considered it to be an addiction. This may not be true for other smokers. I believe that if a person believes a practice to be harmful to him then that possibility exists. *(an unrepentant smoker)*

*****

A week later the results of the tests came in; she [mother] had lung cancer and it had spread to her liver. It was a huge shock for her, and scared her greatly. Then she simply stopped smoking, just like that. (a lifelong nonsmoker)

*****

When I did quit there were withdrawal symptoms, which were very difficult. I enjoy smoking and don't want to quit; cigarettes have been a part of my life for a long time. Smoking is relaxing—it's more enjoyable than eating. I also find that people who smoke seem to be more sociable and friendly. I would like to be able to cut down on the amount I smoke, but haven't even done that. I think it is a habit. I am not sure about addiction. I am not as concerned about dying as I am of being old and sick. (an unrepentant smoker)

*****

I tried to quit within the first year of starting because my husband (boyfriend at that time) abhorred smoking. It was difficult to stop at first, as I was already addicted to tobacco. I would crave cigarettes and certain social situations enhanced my desire to smoke. My boyfriend's strong urging and support made it easier, and gave me the desire to quit. He was a strong reason to quit and with his encouragement I was successful. For several years, however, there were still times when I had a strong desire for a cigarette. You just don't say, "I'm not going to smoke anymore," and stop the need. It takes willpower, time, encouragement, and support from others. (a former smoker)

*****

When I did quit I went through months of drowsiness or boredom. It was difficult to obtain much taste or fragrance satisfaction without lighting a cigarette. Restraining urges to satisfy the pleasure and taste of smoking was tough. Physically, it seemed to me that my metabolism became slower without cigarettes. For several months it seemed that I needed to sleep much more and I was sleepier during my normal waking hours. (a former smoker)

*****

*****

I'm glad I finally realized that if I didn't quit, it would quit me. Myself, my family and my home have never been better. Now when I can, I try to help others, but you have to be careful. I've had some feedback, been told to mind my own business. (a former smoker)

*****

I was really glad to have a good enough reason to quit: to save my life. I went to another doctor who told me to quit and I did; I quit for my family and for me. I feel so good now I will never ever smoke and be a slave to cigarettes again. It was hard to quit—six long months of withdrawal, but I felt better every day. I was finally in control. That's the key word, CONTROL. *Down with tobacco; save our children. Now I hint at everyone else to quit. I probably would have had a heart attack if I had not quit. Cigarettes affected my life for too long. (a former smoker)*

*****

Eleven years after graduation the problems began; I had smoked for about sixteen to seventeen years. I started having difficult bouts with pleurisy and bronchitis, both of which recurred with increasing frequency. Now my family, friends, and doctor really pressured me to quit. It seemed that in the public's eye, smokers were the scum of the earth. No-smoking policies were adopted everywhere, and I began seriously thinking about quitting. I didn't want to be seen as "scum of the earth," and I was concerned about my health. The turning point came when I visited a friend's father in the hospital—he was dying of lung and bone cancer caused by cigarettes. I was horrified—he weighed 100 pounds or less, and looked like he was already dead. He died two days after my visit. I woke up the day after visiting him and decided that it would be the day I quit smoking. I smoked my last cigarette that morning at 7 and told myself to remember it, since it would be my last. I put all my cigarettes in the refrigerator and put on a nicotine patch. (a former smoker)

*****

I'm fifty-three years old. I smoked for about thirty years until I had my first heart attack. If I had known the actual consequences of smoking I would have quit years ago, but I ignored those who kept encouraging me to quit. (a former smoker)

*****

I smoked for ten years before I ever tried to quit. I tried to quit because of my mother. I made the decision to quit not for my sake but hers. It didn't work. All the physical and mental anguish you go through, you can't go through for somebody else. It has to be your decision to quit; you are the one that has to go through it. I have tried to quit smoking three times unsuccessfully. I guess I wasn't really ready to quit—I enjoyed smoking too much. Finally, I decided to quit for myself. I went to a support group for smokers. The people were very honest. They told me that it would be difficult to quit, and that if I broke down and had a cigarette I should not let the guilt beat me down. They told me it was all right to have a cigarette if the feelings got too intense. I must have been ready to quit, because after that meeting I quit cold turkey. I had a very hard time when I quit. I was physically sick for two weeks. Other people I have talked to who also quit did not have the physical sickness and the psychological and emotional turmoil that I did. I consider myself very lucky because the difficulty reinforced my determination to quit. I saw myself, knew I was hooked, and didn't like what I saw. The first five days without cigarettes were a breeze. Then I started to get headaches. Sick to my stomach. Chills. After that the emotional upheaval took over. I would pick fights with my husband and drive him out of the house. Then I would feel guilty and cry for hours. I was a mess. That's when I knew for sure I had been hooked, and I decided I was never going to be hooked again. I knew I was never going to turn into that person again. Nothing I took was going to turn me into that person. Quitting smoking is the hardest thing to do because it is an addiction—not only a physical addiction, but a psychological addiction. It has been over three years since I quit. Smokers have a hard road to travel. You have to remember that smoking is legal. I don't believe anyone should be trying to stop others from smoking in their presence. If the room is well ventilated there is no need to treat cigarette smokers as lepers. That's exactly the way we treat them. Now they have passed legislation so that the only public place they can smoke is outside. I feel bad for them. Quitting smoking is hard enough, but then you have to deal with people harassing you. It's not right. (a former smoker)

*****

For the past two to three years I have tried to quit—I switched to lower tar and nicotine brands and reduced the number of cigarettes I smoked in a day. I got down to one cigarette a day for six months then I started up again, but for two years I kept my intake to less than ten a day. I wanted to quit only because I knew it was bad for my health; I suffered from bronchitis frequently. The most difficult part for me was to tell myself I had to quit because I truly enjoyed it; even now wish I were still smoking. I miss it: the taste, the action, the relaxation. I have to constantly tell myself that it's for my own good that I not smoke. (a former smoker)

*****

I quit in July of 1982. I had three cigarettes left and was thinking about going out and buying another pack for the morning when President Ronald Reagan came on the news saying the tobacco industry was going to get more subsidies, and that they were cutting back on research money for lung cancer. All of a sudden I got mad and yelled at the TV, "You sons of bitches have had me all my life, and you just lost me. I'll never smoke a cigarette again." I called Ronald Reagan every kind of name imaginable, rotten crummy son-of-a-bitch, for taking money from research, the poor and disabled, the near poor, and the soon to be near, near poor. I have not smoked for many years and I have our fearless leader to thank for it. Wasn't that nice of him to stir me up? I was able to quit cold turkey in the end, but I have had no luck getting anyone else to try it. Anger drove me to quit. I was mad at Ronald Reagan for supplying tobacco companies with money, cutting back on research for lung cancer, and leaving the poor and disabled to fall through the net … Anger pumps the adrenaline and cortisone in the body, and that drives my determination in everything I do. It worked on me to quit a habit that I really enjoyed. (a former smoker)

*****

I smoked my last cigarette nineteen years ago in the waiting room as I waited to see if my pregnancy test was positive or negative. It was not very difficult for me to quit. The incentive of having a healthy baby was much greater than the desire to smoke. (a former smoker)

*****

Trying to quit when everyone else around you smokes and you have no place to go is hard. In prison it was really tough. The withdrawals were painful. I was edgy and nervous. I was addicted. Even when I was almost out of money I would spend it on cigarettes instead of food. When I quit I actually developed an eating disorder; I ate to replace smoking. I ended up with a thirty-six-inch waist—picked up about thirty pounds. I quit in June of 1991. I haven't had two cigarettes since. Now, after going on a crusade to ban smoking in the prison, I have become somewhat of a dirty taste in other people's mouths. After I quit I filed an injunction in Federal Court ordering the prison to place me in a nonsmoking area. The prison does not have a nonsmoking area, and I'm now in Federal Court suing the the Department of Corrections to open a nonsmoking unit. The prison staff has labeled me a "nit-picker" and a "troublemaker."

*****

About ten years before I finally quit I was smoking two packs a day. Canadian packs hold twenty-five cigarettes. The cost of cigarettes in Canada has caused many to quit; recently they cost up to $6.80 per pack (today $13.00)—$50.00 a carton. (a former smoker)

*****

Over the years I became addicted to cigarettes, thinking they were enjoyable. As I got older I watched relatives and friends succumb to lung cancer and it set off an alarm in my brain. Attempting several times to quit smoking, I found that I actually craved cigarettes and nicotine. My body would scream out at me, "Hey! You better not deprive me of nicotine!" (a former smoker)

*****

I suppose I'd known for several years that I was addicted to tobacco and was trying forms of behavior modification to lessen the number of cigarettes I smoked. Periodically I quit for a month or two and then resumed smoking five to ten cigarettes per day. I stopped buying cigarettes by the carton and would buy two packages at a time, then one, trying to make it last. I would not allow smoking in my home or automobile. This was mainly a device to help me reduce my own smoking. I did not smoke in my children's homes because of the grandchildren. Again, this was a ploy to help me smoke less. I always followed the no-smoking laws: I always felt it was one less cigarette I smoked. (a former smoker)

*****

I try to tell people there is only one way: cold turkey. That's what I did. It takes a little effort but it works fine and it's free. (a former smoker)

*****

I first wanted to quit about fifteen years after I started smoking. It took me another fifteen years to accomplish this feat. Of course, you realize right away within the first or second year of smoking that it is not good for you, but you don't realize you are hooked already—you just laugh it off and keep smoking. The most difficult part of quitting was failing at it. What I did was, I'd light a cigarette, take two or three drags, realize I didn't want to smoke, that I didn't want the cigarette, and so end up throwing it away. I learned to throw the cigarettes in a water-filled container, setting up empty tin cans as ashtrays for this purpose, so I could not re-light them. I found I didn't buy any more cigarettes per day, and that I was smoking way, way less. This made me feel positive; I had regained control over my habit. I have given this idea to other smokers who say they'd like to quit, or are trying to but have so far had no luck. (a former smoker)

*****

As time went on, I began to suffer from allergies and respiratory problems until I finally realized that smoking was causing me a lot of problems. So, I quit "cold turkey" and have not smoked one cigarette since then. (a former smoker)

*****

I was addicted to the entire concept of smoking, not just the nicotine. When I quit I wore no patch and had few symptoms of nicotine withdrawal. I believe this is an individual matter. I miss all the motions and comforts of smoking, not the taste, smell or nicotine effects. I did not go to a restaurant or bar for six weeks after I quit, and I still have trouble playing bridge without my cigarettes. Quitting is like losing your best friend. It changed my life. Now I drink very little and do not go bar hopping or just sit around and drink and chat with people. I have to be doing something, and I couldn't handle the alcohol without cigarettes—they just went together for me. I gained fifteen pounds over the first year before I changed my eating habits and started exercising regularly. Another lifestyle change! When I smoked I kept my ideal weight with little thought; when others ate, I smoked. I miss that, but I adjusted my habits over time. It was not easy. I consider quitting to be one of the greatest accomplishments of my life. I expected that I would miss cigarettes forever, and tried to take it one day at a time. I admitted to everyone that it was hard for me. I was patient with myself and accepted that it was hard work and, for the first several months, all consuming. The desire to smoke will always be there. You have to change your lifestyle, routine, and habits in order to quit. Once I acknowledged the power tobacco had over me, everything was easier. Acknowledging that I was not in control was the hardest—I accepted that the day I quit. I knew I was really addicted the year before I quit, when I tried to play games with myself to reduce use and/or change habits. It would work for awhile and then I'd be right back to a pack a day. I loved smoking. I enjoyed it. And I was always addicted. I tell everyone who asks how I did it that "You must acknowledge your addiction and live with it every day." It's been six years and I still occasionally wish I could have a smoke, but I choose not to. I try not to push others, but I am very supportive of those who have quit or want to quit. (a former smoker)

*****

When I try to quit, it goes fine at the start because of my willpower and sense of determination. However, at the first sign of stress or temptation to alcohol, I become emotionally weak; my strength to resist then deteriorates quickly. I did, however, quit two times—during both of my pregnancies. I did not or could not harm the life growing inside of me. After the births, however, I resumed smoking. It's hard to say why exactly—just a nagging inside my head that I needed to resume. When I try to cut back every so often, I think of all the money I put into the habit. Once a year I get a bad case of bronchitis; I know that smoking may not cause it, but I know it doesn't help it get better. When I do cut back, these are the withdrawal symptoms: headache, vomiting spells, irritability, nervousness, and impatience. Also, I am afraid of gaining weight. (a smoker who can't quit)

*****

Like alcoholism, the incentive to quit has to come from within. I never believed that outside pressure would work—it makes you feel guilty and resentful of the pressure. In my experience, that pressure often leads to secret smoking. The longing for a cigarette was the most difficult part of quitting, especially after a meal, with tea, coffee or a drink. During times of either stress or anger, I would reach for a cigarette. Just the idea of a cigarette made me salivate long after I did quit. I still occasionally think about having a cigarette; however, if I did inhale I know that it would be anything but pleasant—I have no fear of ever trying it again. (a former smoker)

*****

What was difficult about quitting? Wanting it; dreaming of smoking; seeing other people smoke; and gaining weight. It was so hard to stop thinking about smoking and so easy to start after just one. (an unrepentant smoker)

*****

I tried many times to quit without success after my mother died. Her death made me want to quit and I did after many attempts. I think the biggest hurdle was convincing myself that I had to quit. Once I had completely convinced myself, I was able to do it and lost the desire to smoke altogether. I quit when I actually realized I was killing myself. I was killing myself making the tobacco industry rich, along with millions of other smokers. (a former smoker)

*****

I quit cold turkey in 1951. My wife and two children hated the smell and the effects of the smoke. I began to cough and produce phlegm. During withdrawal from tobacco I had all the symptoms of addiction withdrawal: tension and nerves, loss of ability to taste, loss of appetite, weight loss, aches and pains—especially in the back and chest—and coughing. Money was a factor, too. When I quit I had a wife, two kids and was in debt; I couldn't afford to smoke. I advised all my smoking patients to stop and save the money for education or insurance. Some did, others promised to quit "someday." If they quit they were very thankful. Others said, "I can afford to keep doing it." (a former smoker)

*****

I am a forty-five-year-old widow with two wonderful sons, a Master's degree in education, a great job, and a thirty-year habit that's killing my spirit and probably my body. At times I feel overwhelmed by my addiction and all of its ramifications. As I write this, I am going through pure hell—again; it has been two months and three days since my last cigarette. I have quit many times: once for a year, once for nine months and numerous other times for shorter periods. Why is smoking so repugnant that I put myself through the siege of quitting time after time? It makes me feel crazy. There, I said it, and I guess that really is the bottom line. My husband died from cancer eight years ago, so for me to smoke in front of my two children is almost unforgivable. They worry with good reason that I'll die of cancer. I worry about the second-hand smoke thing, that they'll be more apt to take up smoking themselves. I play these scenarios in my head every time I inhale. (a smoker who can't quit)

*****

I can't say exactly what caused me to quit precisely six months ago at forty-nine. My health seemed all right, but because of my age, I began to get concerned for my health. I wasn't sure about my hay fever condition and I heard "propaganda" that smoking increases respiratory problems for older people, but I didn't know what to believe. The prospect of my Navy retirement was perhaps one factor. This was a major life adjustment. Also, laws against smoking in public buildings limited my smoke breaks. Often it was too cold to go outside or too inconvenient since I was on an extremely hectic schedule at all hours because of my relocation. Some of my coworkers began joining nonsmoking clinics. People talked more about the fact that it was NOT cool to smoke. All these events coincided with the momentous anniversary of my father's death. (a former smoker)

*****

At forty-six my doctor told me if I didn't quit smoking I would get emphysema and I'd probably die in five years. I had gone to her for bronchitis. I told my husband and he said, "You can't quit if I keep smoking." He, God bless him, put out his last cigarette and hasn't smoked since; he was forty-eight. I realized I was addicted when I was about forty-five. Addiction is most pleasurable. Your body screams for that nicotine hit. I tried reducing the cigarettes I smoked daily, but that didn't work. My husband, children, grandchildren and sisters, nephews, and nieces tried to help me quit. Finally, I was so sick I went to another no-smoking class and told my husband before I went that he would never see me smoke again. I smoked my last cigarette January 8, 1993, at sixty- three. Thank God! (a former smoker)

*****

When we married, Frank and I both smoked. He smoked up to three packs a day, and I smoked between one and two packs a day. Within the first year of our marriage, I contracted bronchitis three times and coughed constantly. My doctor said that "If you get this one more time and if you're still smoking, don't come back to me." That's when I knew I had to quit. My last cigarette was in June of l969; it was the most difficult thing I have ever done. I have not had bronchitis or even a bad cold since. (a former smoker)

*****

I prayed to God and took an oath on the Bible. Over the next several weeks I was guided from within on how to change my lifestyle patterns, such as substituting juice for coffee and eating lunch outside instead of in the break room. My fear of breaking an oath to God sustained me; I managed to finally quit. Today, twenty-five years later, I can say I have never smoked again. Once in a while though, I still dream I am smoking. (a former smoker)

*****

I did manage to quit from 1983 to 1985 and gained thirty pounds, which I have never been able to lose since. I quit using self-induced psychology, something I don't seem able to repeat. I believe that the entrapment is ninety percent psychological and only ten percent nicotine-related. I was a fool to start again in 1985—one cigarette did it. I thought that I could by then "take them or leave them." I feel like a pest, a weakling and an ignoramus! (a smoker who can't quit)

*****

My wife of forty-six years doesn't smoke, and neither do my three grown children. None of them have ever smoked. In the past few years I tried a number of times to cut down on my smoking. In fact, I tried to stop smoking about five years ago. I suffered from severe withdrawal symptoms—I kept insisting it was the "flu." After about five days I started smoking my pipe again. During the last several years I have tried to cut down on my smoking out of respect for my family. I have also stopped smoking in the house and in our vehicles; I went on a lot of long walks. In February of 1993 I went for a medical check-up after not having had a thorough check-up for over five years. I knew something was wrong when the lab phoned me and asked when I last had my chest x-rayed. The doctor told me I had a shadow on my right lung! I subsequently had more x-rays and a CAT scan and was sent to a surgeon. He informed me that there was no way of determining just what this shadow was unless I had surgery. I think that it was at this point that I wished I had never smoked, that they had thrown all the tobacco in the ocean, and that we had never heard of Sir Walter Raleigh. I quit smoking. I became very nervous and agitated during withdrawal and had to consult my family doctor for something to calm me down and help me sleep. (a former smoker)

*****

If I knew about the actual impurities in tobacco twenty years ago I would have quit then! I didn't know until 1993 that more than 4,000 chemical compounds have been identified in tobacco smoke, at least forty-three of which are known to cause cancer in humans. Plus, each year secondhand smoke kills over 3,000 adult nonsmokers from lung cancer. (a former smoker)

*****

Probably the hardest part, after the first few days of withdrawal, is just breaking habits: When I pick up the phone, I light a cigarette; when I start the dishwasher, I light a cigarette; when I get a drink of coffee or whatever, I light a cigarette and I light a cigarette every time I start the car. I don't know what to do with my hands. Teenagers can't comprehend just how hard it is to quit smoking. They have no idea that they are taking on a lifelong problem. (a smoker who can't quit)

*****

I tried to quit or cut back because my ex-husband resented the amount of money I spent on cigarettes. I also tried to quit or cut back because I was hospitalized with a lung ailment. I have tried to quit and cut back, and I have been forced to do so because of social stigma, smoking bans, and a lack of opportunity to smoke. Smoking is such an integral part of my work habits that I find I can't think without smoking—especially in stressful work situations. Smoking is also such an integral part of my socializing, especially when I drink. It's also very enjoyable at the end of a meal. I crave cigarettes, period. I'm addicted. I can't go more than two hours comfortably without a cigarette. Addiction is hell. It is a craving in the throat for satisfaction, nervousness, fidgeting, tenseness and irritability. It is uppermost and paramount in my consideration of going somewhere on what mode of transportation: Will I be able to smoke?

I never even leave the house without checking to see that I have my cigarettes, lighter and ashtray, and I get very disturbed if I discover I don't have my cigarettes with me. Just having them with me is sometimes enough. Hell is realizing at midnight that I have no more cigarettes. Hell is realizing you're in a situation where you won't be able to smoke for hours and hours, such as in airplane or train travel. It is very unpleasant to have to continually justify, rationalize and defend your habit and to despise yourself for weakness when millions of others have managed to quit. I avoid the doctor because I know I will get harangued about smoking. I fear "when that day comes to pay the piper for smoking for so many years." I fear the possibility of a terrible death and being unable to quit. (a smoker who can't quit)

*****

I have tried many times to quit and have quit for up to a few weeks. The first time being maybe two years after I started. I tried to quit because of the increasing awareness of its ill effects on long-term health. I always seemed to give in because people around me smoked. I guess the most difficult part is to give up the habit of having a cigarette in your hand, and the nicotine withdrawal. I think it is a nervous habit for me and I don't know how to fix that situation. When I tried to quit I realized that it had become an addiction, because I was very nervous and irritable without cigarettes. However, when I got through the first few days I was okay until something stressful happened that I couldn't cope with without a cigarette. Once I did quit, I told others that it would help me to abstain if they would not smoke in my presence. (a smoker who can't quit)

*****

If I didn't have cigarettes I would lose my temper very easily, and my girlfriend and I came close to breaking up because of these times. Smoking is almost as bad as alcohol. It can destroy a relationship almost as easily. I first tried to quit when I was twenty-three…two summers ago when I tried out for a baseball team I realized I hadn't been as active as I used to be. My smoking was affecting me, so I just decided to quit "cold turkey." While in withdrawal, every time somebody would smoke in front of me I would be tempted to smoke, but I would instead make them smoke away from me. I finally gave it up, but I was very frustrated and took it all out on my girlfriend and immediate family. (a smoker who can't quit)

*****

For other addictions, daily outpatient help is provided. Quitting smoking means a complete change of lifestyle. In my opinion, the lifestyle change is greater for smokers than alcohol or drug addicts. However, the same understanding and help isn't available for tobacco addicts...Smokers are treated like weak outcasts by many, instead of people with an addictive habit that many of us ourselves despise. Nonsmokers do not understand on the whole, and we choose our friends and social life by our habit. Most of us try to be considerate, but we are still ostracized. This does not help us when we really do not like our dependency either...I would very much like to be a nonsmoker, but it is very difficult after so many years. It affects who my friends are and my social life. (a smoker who can't quit)

*****

The most difficult part of quitting or cutting back on tobacco is trying not to think about it. I would leave home to run an errand and leave my tobacco "life vest" behind—this took extreme bravery. Though tense and anxious while gone, I managed to survive. Right now, I can't bring myself to do that—I make sure I have my wallet, keys, and double check to make sure I have my cigarettes whenever I leave home. (a smoker who can't quit)

*****

I first tried to quit at twenty-two. I had no problems, but four weeks later started again and had to try to quit again a year later. The second time was a bear, for some reason. I had quite a struggle emotionally—my husband and I had gone through a divorce. The first lime I quit for no reason. The second time, because God told me to. I had been using cigarettes as an emotional substitute. The cigarette was my "friend," and now it was gone. I didn't know what to do with my hands. I had no "props" when I spoke to people. I became more and more introverted, but all the ex-smokers I knew told me it would help my body if I quit, and God told me to, so I forced myself to abstain. (a former smoker)

*****

Every day I try to quit and always fail. The more I think about quitting, the faster I smoke! I have asked God's help, asked that He take away my desire and need to smoke. The only help other people give is, "Just quit..." and, "You're not trying hard enough." I have also turned to my doctor and myself.

I have been given Nicorette to chew and nicotine patches—all to no avail. I smoked while using them. The patches did reduce my smoking somewhat. Nicorette did nothing for me. (a smoker who can't quit)

*****

Quitting is tough! Especially losing the physical aspect of smoking: no longer being able to reach for, light, and then smoke a cigarette for distraction, to occupy your thoughts, time and hands. Smoking gives you an out when you need a moment away from a situation to relax or regroup. I use smoking as an exercise to take a break from work or writing. The act of smoking and its comforting, familiar presence remains for a long, long time. (a smoker who can't quit)

Stories

I Feel Like a Pest, a Weakling, and an Ignoramus!—A Smoker Who Can't Quit

I really would like to be free of the tyranny of tobacco; I'd like to be able to "take it or leave it."

I can tell the damage smoking for more than fifty years has done to me. I often have lung congestion, and when I awake in the middle of the night or early morning, I cough up phlegm. My ability to walk fast is also impaired.

Tobacco use will definitely affect my future. I have been a strong, robust person for most of my life. I felt like my body was good for more than ninety years, but if I can't stop smoking I'm afraid I might not get past seventy-five. I don't mind dying, but I don't relish the thought of a painful, lingering illness before death. Also, I don't want to leave my wife a widow. I also worry about being hospitalized and not being able to smoke.

I started smoking at sixteen in high school; I wanted to be a "regular guy" and smoke like all the other "guys." Father was a smoker and wouldn't allow me to smoke till I was sixteen. At first, I smoked to feel "big." It was WWII that set it in concrete; I was in heavy combat, so when I was able to rest and smoke it was the world's greatest comfort, next to still being alive. Today, the taste, mildness, and menthol attract me to smoke.

My spouse smokes. Our friends are opposed to my smoking and to smoking in general; therefore, I can't be with them for long without leaving them to go out for a smoke. This puts a damper on friendships.

Every day I try to quit and always fail. The more I think about quitting, the faster I smoke! I have asked God's help, asked that He take away my desire and need to smoke. Smoking temporarily satisfies my craving. I also like to browse in tobacco shops, there's a mystique to them. I like pipes and cigars too, but I love cigarettes the best. It's mainly necessary as a "fix," but it's also enjoyable when relaxing.

My addiction is such that about every fifty minutes or so I feel a strong urge to have one—throughout the day. I usually go to bed at about ten and wake up at about four to go to the bathroom, and then I have to have a cigarette. If I'm with company, I can usually hold out for a couple of hours. The most difficult part of quitting or cutting back on tobacco is trying not to think about it.

If they raised taxes on tobacco products as a way to discourage tobacco use, I would do poorly; I would still buy them. I think it's unfair when they don't also raise the tax on fast food products and include restaurants and pastry shops, which contribute to clogging the arteries. They should also penalize motorcyclists, surfboarders, waterskiers, skateboarders, and people who lay out in the sun getting sunburned. And what about alcohol?

My Whole Adult Life Has Revolved Around Smoking—A Smoker Who Can't Quit

I strongly believe that my addiction to nicotine began at birth in 1957. I believe that I was born with a genetic predisposition to smoke. Both my parents were smokers, and my mother was an alcoholic. All of my uncles and many aunts smoked. My older sisters smoked when they became teenagers. All my parents' friends smoked and as I became a teenager so did my friends.

My first experience with smoking was at an early experimental stage with my brother and friends. All our parents smoked. Cigarettes were always readily available in fancy cigarette boxes around the house. We would smoke to look, act, and play like grown-ups. We were raised with cigarette advertising all around us—the Marlboro Man, "You've Come a Long Way Baby," and others. Women were sophisticated, elegant, and "sexy" if they smoked.

I began smoking seriously at sixteen. I had moved to Long Island from a small town in southern New Jersey; I was very lonely and had put on a great deal of weight—I was miserable. I made friends with peers who smoked, and after my many days of "trying" cigarettes at a younger age, I knew how to do it well—it was easy. My mother allowed me to smoke in the house because she knew I would anyway. She bought me cigarettes, and I purchased them myself at local stores; getting cigarettes was never a problem.

My smoking continued throughout high school, although in the late 1970s many of my friends had either quit or were nonsmokers. Unfortunately, I had been smoking long enough that it was now very difficult to stop. I didn't smoke when I was with that group of friends. I was also involved with many athletic groups, church groups, and family activities, and I dated a smoker. I monitored my smoking accordingly.

In college, I had a tougher time because then smoking was really not the thing to do (1978–1979). We were allowed to smoke in the dorms and at the cafeteria, however, so I managed to continue with my addiction. On my first trip to Alaska in 1977, I realized that smoking would be a barrier in my future. Smokers there were in a class by themselves—the lowest of low—and really not tolerated. I still managed to find a way, and mostly smoked alone.

After graduation in 1979, I moved to Alaska to begin my teaching career. I was dating a man at the time who was very much a nonsmoker. I only smoked outdoors or when he wasn't around. Our relationship soon ended. I then met my husband and we dated for over a year. He is a smoker. We have been married now for twelve years.

Because I am a teacher, I spend a great deal of time trying to convince young people to avoid using any drug that might damage their physical or emotional health. I feel I am a passionate speaker on this topic because of my own problems with addiction.

Shortly after I began teaching fifteen years ago, our school district began designated smoking areas. They were always the smallest, least ventilated, unattractive "cells," until finally smoking was barred altogether. That was a real eye-opener for me; my life changed drastically. I didn't fully realize the extent of my addiction until I was no longer able to smoke at school.

Before the ban, I arrived at work around 7:30 a.m. and left at around 6:00 p.m. I did all my planning, organizing, and much of my grading before and after school. Then, I only had to bring home a few things to finish. After the ban, I wouldn't arrive at work until 8 a.m. and always left at 4 p.m. I also left campus at noon to smoke after lunch. Over the last five years, two of my smoking friends at work have quit. I am alone. In just these last eight weeks, I have quit going out at noon. My colleagues were very helpful and supportive of me in my effort to quit. I have been at work as long as nine hours without smoking.

Earlier, I saw doctors for my addiction problems. I seriously considered counseling, but my medical program covers only fifty percent of ten sessions. Each session is $120 with an initial session of $150. I cannot afford to pay for the balance, and our medical insurance does not cover nicotine dependence counseling, patches, gum, or any other wellness kind of program.

Within the last three weeks, I have been diagnosed with a medical problem that may require surgery and have been told to quit smoking. I'm not sure which I fear more, quitting or surgery. My whole adult life has revolved around smoking. Evert habit, relationship, crisis, decision, lifestyle choice have revolved around smoking. Cigarettes have been my "best friend" and my worst enemy. Cigarettes are my stress outlet, my calming mechanism, my stimulant, and my relaxant. They are part of everything I do every day from getting up in the morning to sleeping at night. I have attempted quitting three times, once successfully for three weeks. I returned though because I want to be a smoker more than I want to be a nonsmoker. I don't know myself as a nonsmoker and don't know that I want to.

Today, however, I'm not sure what I want. As I was telling a friend recently, I don't think I've ever been more afraid in my life. I told my doctor I would need more than just a patch to quit smoking. I don't know what I'll do. I stand at a major crossroads.

I truly wish I had never started smoking. I ache for the teenagers I see start every day. I wish cigarettes were illegal—and no longer available. I just finished teaching a unit on Colonial America. It is ironic to think that our country was basically founded on the cash crop of tobacco, among other things of course. If we only knew then…

I don't have any answers, only questions. I don't want to blame others, for ultimately it was my choice that put me where I am today. I just wonder how all this will turn out.

I Feel Very Befuddled and I Really Miss My Cigarettes— A Smoker Who Can't Quit

I started smoking many years ago while working at a major hotel in New York City. Judy, the mail clerk, smoked. Every day she would offer me a cigarette and one day I took one, and then another, until I felt obligated to buy a pack to repay her. We would smoke together—her out of need and me to keep up. I didn't smoke alone back in those years, and I only smoked at work.

I grew up with a nonsmoking family. I felt no need or desire to smoke. At the age of twenty-three, I should have known better. Of course, we were not educated about smoking as we are today. I did not know at the time that I was setting up myself for an addiction.

When I became pregnant with my second child, for three months I became ill if I smoked or was near smoke. In the fourth or fifth month, I was able to smoke again and enjoyed it. Doctors did not warn us against smoking back then.

It's hard to convince my children not to smoke when I'm still smoking myself. We can't let go of it. Both my sons smoke. They do not feel good about it and are feeling the effects. I suppose in a way I taught them to smoke when they were still at home. One was born a premature baby; he has many respiratory problems. Smoking also bothers my youngest son.

I did not make very many good choices for myself over the years. Husband #1 smoked, drank heavily, and was abusive. Husband #2 had many addictions, but smoking was not one of them. Because I did not know any better, I chose a path of destruction. Husband #2 nagged me quite a bit about smoking, but I needed my friendly cigarettes, needed that addictive crutch to get by. I never really had what you would call a stable home life. In smoking, I found something that I could count on and control, and no one was going to take that away.

Husband #3 drinks and smokes heavily. Needless to say, my third choice of spouse is as bad as the first two. Again, smoking is my best friend.

I developed breast cancer. I had seven weeks of radiation and in the end the breast had to be removed. I know my lung must be badly scarred from the radiation—the skin on the front and back was badly burned. The doctor has asked me many times to quit smoking, and

I keep trying without success. I have tried everything suggested except for Habitrol patches. For some reason, they scare me.

I buy one pack a day; if I bought a carton, I would smoke ten packs a week instead of seven. I tried buying cigarettes that were on sale—cheap ones. They would hurt my lungs, so I went back to the lowest tar and nicotine cigarettes: one milligram of nicotine and one milligram of tar.

Yesterday morning, a bee stung me close to my eye. In the late afternoon, I stopped at the doctor's since I had to go grocery shopping anyway; the area around my eye was swollen and hurting; and I had a terrible headache. I was given a tetanus shot, a flu shot since I was there, a prescription for infection and Benadryl. I had a cigarette at midnight. It is now 2:45 p.m. Thursday afternoon and I haven't had a cigarette since going to bed at midnight and only because I don't feel well. The nurse gave me some patches to try out this morning. I didn't put one on. Like I said, for some reason they scare me more than my smoking does.

I am a nervous wreck today—due to a lack of nicotine, I suppose. I feel very befuddled and really miss my cigarettes. I guess when I go home at 4:30 p.m., I will have one to get me settled down. It makes me angry that I let smoking control me. I thought that this was the one thing in my life I controlled—how wrong I was. Now that smoking is considered unacceptable, I feel quite guilty when I light up in front of someone. All it does is add to the list of things to feel guilty about, not to mention the fear of damage to my own health. I wish there were some easy way to quit and get back to feeling like I did when I was a nonsmoker. I can discipline myself with other things in my life, but not smoking.

My sister is coming to visit. Tomorrow when she comes downstairs, she won't be able to breathe because of the smoke from my husband and me. I am going to try to be a considerate smoker while she and her husband are here. We have lost many friends who quit smoking; they can't stand being around a smoky house and people smelling of smoke. I remember back years ago when I felt the same way.

So, even my two bouts with cancer have not stopped this terrible habit. It's pretty scary to know I have an addiction that with such a powerful hold on me. Also, I am worried about all the children and other people who do not deserve to be affected by our second-hand smoke.

I feel we should be free to choose if we want to smoke or not, but I also feel that nonsmokers should not be subjected to our smoke invading their lungs and saturating their clothes.

We smoke because we once chose to, and now we smoke because we haven't the willpower to stop.

Postscript

My sister and her husband have come and gone. I was a considerate smoker only because I was still ill from the bee sting. I was smoking only two cigarettes a day because I needed a nicotine fix. Three days ago, I started wearing the patch to see if I could kick this rotten addiction. I put it on in the morning and I had to pull it off at about 6 p.m. because my heart felt like it would run away and the patch hurt. Usually, I need to smoke one cigarette every morning around nine. Today I fought that desire. It is now close to noon and I'm still fighting. This is the first time I have felt like really fighting it for any length of time, and I can see that I'm in for a very rough time. My nerves are frazzled, my body is tense, and my mind befuddled. In my head, I have a vision of cigarettes. I want one and it's all I can think about. My body craves that cigarette and my mind must fight my desire. I pray and hope that I can make it. Even with a serious illness knocking at my door, this fight is extremely hard.

After All These Years I Thought I Was Safe from Addiction—A Smoker Who Can't Quit

One scorching summer afternoon while reclining on a torn down cornstalk at the age of thirteen, I had my first cigarette. It wasn't an after-sex smoke; we were smoking from a pack that my fellow worker had lifted out of her mom's purse before starting for work that morning. We had "arrived." We were "cool." We rested and puffed, coughed, and puffed again. After a while, the little white stick seemed friendlier, until it became an anxiously awaited treat at the end of each row of corn. We continued until the pack lay limp on the ground at the end of the day. My introduction lasted only that one day, but the memory lingered, and in the summer of my eighteenth birthday, I tried again. I don't know why I waited those five years, but I did.

In early summer, I was hired for a couple of weeks to tend a lovely eighty-five-year-old woman while her daughter worked. The daughter who hired me smoked, and each day while the old woman napped, I lifted a slender white cigarette from the dainty box on the coffee table and went into the bathroom to converse with the mirror. It was very "in" to smoke in those days, and I wanted to make sure the young woman in the mirror did it right. I practiced holding it properly. I practiced inhaling and exhaling, all the while making certain my image remained chic and ladylike. At the end of my tour of duty I was hooked, although I didn't realize it then. When I returned to my summer cornfield job in August, I had graduated to toting my own pack of 100s.

Dad smoked; mother didn't. I was too shy to face my family with my new adventure, so when I wanted a cigarette at home I went into the bathroom, opened the window and lit up. Sometimes, I used the rubber plug from the bathtub as an ashtray. I always sprayed room deodorant generously and left the window open when exiting—I didn't fool anyone!

After attending a crash course at my hometown college, I found myself teaching—it was my first time away from home. All the teachers in the school smoked and the air in our private coffee room was choked with the stench of constant use.

Semesters grew into years and the years eventually led me to the great land of sunshine—California. Lacking enough college time to teach in California, I was thrown into corporate employment. After 11 years, I noticed that my endurance had dwindled a bit; it was nothing drastic, but as I was athletic, it seemed a warning. I decided to stop smoking. I bought a huge bag of hard candies and threw away my cigarettes. Perhaps I had stronger will in those days; perhaps the timing was just right. Whatever the reason, it worked. I didn't touch a cigarette for eight years. There were times when I'd have done anything for a smoke, but I didn't. The sweet smell that arose when someone lit up nearly drove me crazy several times, but I still didn't smoke.

In the fall of 1973, my life turned some terrible flip-flops, and in one particularly precarious moment, I bummed a cigarette. I thought I was safe from addiction—clearly, I wasn't. This one cigarette led me to buy my own and there I was, right back where I had started.

I am still puffing away. In the past ten years, I have been hypnotized four times for smoking. Each time freed me from my addiction for only a month or two. I've been pin-cushioned by two different acupuncturists to no avail, and I have seen a therapist specializing in smoke therapy twice; the latter worked for a couple of months. I have "quit" for twenty-three days cold turkey on my own only to take a cigarette a friend offered; of course, I started smoking again.

Today, I feel a huge sense of defeat. What was once the curious lark of a thirteen-year-old girl in Nebraska has led to the bitter defeat of a middle-aged California woman. For some reason, I fail to rustle up that inner determination that I found when I quit for those eight years so long ago. I tell myself all the preaching about the dangers of smoking that I know to be true, but it doesn't work! I throw a pack away one day only to buy a replacement the next.

There is a glimmer of hope, however. Last week, I met with my sister for a few days. We stayed in a nonsmoking hotel and I had to slip out to have my "fix." My sister is very special. She never criticizes me, but she's never smoked and I know she worries about me, as do my whole family of nonsmokers. Late the last night, we were there I excused myself just before bedtime to go outside for a cigarette. It was such a major undertaking that by the time I got back up to our room I was ready for another smoke! As I left our room for the second time, I glanced back at my sister and said something like, "Isn't it terrible?" I saw the look in her eyes as she answered, "I just feel so sorry for you." I've thought of that moment ever since, and somehow I've got to try again. I can't bear to hurt those I love any longer. Somewhere I must have the strength to walk away from this addiction.

I Hate the Fact That I Am Addicted to a Filthy, Dirty Habit—A Smoker Who Can't Quit

I have been a smoker for forty years. At first I was a light smoker. Now I smoke heavily. My younger sister had a heart attack and she still smokes. I try to encourage her to quit—I don't want her to die young of a heart attack. She's lost weight, is getting her cholesterol down, and is smoking less.

I have tried many times myself to quit, but always failed. Once I quit for a year, but recently the longest I have been able to quit has been four weeks. When I do quit, I feel a tremendous loss, gain weight, and feel depressed. I can't try to get my daughter to quit if I can't.

I hate that I'm so addicted to this filthy, dirty habit, and wish I had known before I started that it was so addictive.

I exercise regularly and think how foolish it is to smoke at the same time. For other addictions, daily outpatient help is provided. Quitting smoking means a complete change of lifestyle. In my opinion, the lifestyle change is greater for smokers than for alcohol or drug addicts. However, the same understanding and help are not available for tobacco addicts.

I plan to quit at the beginning of the New Year; I am trying to "psych" myself in the meantime. I wish there were some kind of pill available for smokers that I could take (a physically harmless one) that would make a person nauseated if they tried to light up.

Smokers are treated like weak outcasts by many instead of people with an addictive habit that we ourselves despise.

Nonsmokers are not understanding on the whole, and we choose our friends and social life by our habit. Most of us try to be considerate, but we are still ostracized. This does not help us when we really don't like our dependency either.

I would like very much to be a nonsmoker, but it is very difficult after so many years. It affects my social life and who my friends are. I am not proud to say I'm a smoker. Hopefully, just writing this out will help me overcome my addiction.

I Hate Everything About Smoking, But I Love to Smoke and I Can't Stop!—A Smoker Who Can't Quit

I love smoking; it's been an integral part of my life for thirty-seven years. I am very high strung; smoking soothes me. When I am upset, I can't wait to have a cigarette. If I could either smoke or eat, I would choose to smoke. I don't patronize nonsmoking restaurants, and before I go into a retail store, I smoke so I won't have a "nicotine fit" while I shop.

I can't smoke at work, so I smoke constantly before I go to work, as though I could build up a reserve of nicotine. When work is stressful, all I can think about is a cigarette. I go outside in any kind of weather and have a quick cigarette as soon as I can. I hate standing outside to smoke; it's like being a school kid.

I kept smoking lighter and lighter cigarettes in hope of reducing the health risks, but they satisfy my need for nicotine less and less so I smoke more and more.

I hate smoking; my house smells terrible, my clothes smell terrible… My last car smelled so terrible even I couldn't stand it. I almost never smoke in my new car, so I stop at rest areas to get out and smoke, and I smoke in parking lots while walking to and from the car.

I am getting frightened now because I feel smoking is beginning to affect my health. I have chest discomfort, I'm short of breath, I get bronchitis frequently, and when I get a cold it hangs on for weeks. I always thought I'd quit before I was old. I used to hate to see old women smoking. Time flies; I'm now fifty-five. I look like an old smoker and I'm starting to be afraid I won't live long enough. I have a thirty-six-year-old daughter who is mildly retarded (I can't even think that smoking during my pregnancy was a contributing factor). She needs me. A number of years ago, my doctor asked me when I was going to quit smoking. I quipped, "Probably when it's too late." Now I'm afraid that will be a self-fulfilling prophecy.

I'm starting to feel like a social outcast. I feel like a fool standing out in the freezing cold smoking. I'm smoking now as I write this. I've had eight cigarettes in the past hour since I came home from work. I'm angry that there are so many places you can't smoke, and I'm furious when people are upset about my smoking. I think smokers are to be pitied. I'm angry because my husband thinks I can quit smoking because he did—my smoking is increasingly annoying him. Many of my friends have the same problem with their husbands.

I love a clean house, but I can't keep up with my filthy windows and curtains. Everything in the house is yellow. I hate everything about smoking, but I love to smoke and I just can't stop!

When I started smoking as a teenager, I thought it was sophisticated and daring. My mother hated smoking, which made it even more desirable to me. I thought I could quit at any time.

My husband doesn't know how much I smoke—I will not admit it to him.

Why have I never made a serious effort to quit smoking? Because I love it and don't believe for a second that I can quit. It's how I cope! I think, it is a horrible habit. If only I hadn't started…

I Chased this Guy, Threatening to Brain Him with My Crutches—A Former Smoker

The toughest part about quitting was undergoing surgery for the complete removal of my left lung. This is not a method that I would recommend for smoking-cessation clinics. After seven weeks in critical care, I lost the urge to smoke. In fact, when I encountered smoke from other patients in my ten-week hospital stay, I had paroxysms and spasms that seemed life-threatening. Yes, Virginia, hard as it is to believe, some other lung cancer victims recovering from surgery went right back to smoking as soon as they were off the ventilator! This totally amazed me!

I was in a VA hospital and my roommate had had his leg amputated due, I suspect, to a combination of diabetes and tobacco-induced poor circulation. He insisted on smoking in the room we shared against hospital regulations and my vehement wishes. They called security when they saw me chasing this guy and threatening to brain him with one of my crutches. The only thing that prevented me from doing this was that he was just a bit faster than in his wheelchair than I was on crutches. This began my militancy against tobacco.

I try not to miss the opportunity to tell young people about how tobacco has affected me. Most often I provide them with a VERY graphic description of how a pneumonectomy is performed—with the patient on his side on a table that operates like a garage lift; it elevates the thoracic region by means of a hydraulic lift. Then the body is cut in half, one rib removed and the adjacent rib broken in order for two surgeons to get their hands inside the chest cavity. I have been known to follow this up by removing my shirt to demonstrate the thoracotomy scar; it's vivid and runs from my breastbone to my spine. Three people I spoke to have subsequently quit.

I have told several smoking mothers or babes-in-arms that smoking while holding an infant or smoking in an automobile with a child amounts to child abuse. Tactful? Hell, no—I'm a curmudgeon! If you don't want to hear it, don't do it.

My childhood peers considered me a nerd. I lived in a fairly isolated residential cluster set amidst a small farming community fifteen miles from town. About the only social interaction available was with a neighborhood gang comprised of around twenty-five youths of my age and older. All of these kids were smokers, and a large part or my early smoking was to gain peer-group acceptance. Also, my father, grandfather, my uncle (who lived with us) all smoked, as did my physician, teacher, Episcopal priest, bishop, and local politicians. My president, F.D.R., was seldom seen without his famous cigarette holder. Tobacco advertising was rampant, "Camels—not a cough in a carload." And, "More doctors have switched to Camels than any other brand." Also, "Lucky Strike green has gone to war," alluding to the green printer's ink that went into the package.

It was a powerful habit that I tried to break many, many times, especially when suffering about of pleurisy or bronchitis. Even before all the hoopla about the bad effects, I was very much aware that it was doing me irrevocable harm. "They" say that smokers have low self-esteem—I think, this is a problem that stems from not being in control of one's life enough to be able to quit. That is at least true in my case.

I once enrolled in a quit-smoking program sponsored by one of our local hospitals. Several prominent members of the medical community talked down to the assembly, we were acquainted with celery and carrot sticks, and paired with another group member so that we could call them at any hour of the day or night if we felt we were "losing it." My partner, a middle-aged female junior administrator on the hospital staff was unable to get over her concern over the social implications of calling/receiving odd-hour telephone messages from a member of the opposite sex. The program was a big waste of time, being completely ineffectual for me and for anyone that I talked with. The experience merely reinforced my lack of faith in such an endeavor, no matter how well meaning it might be.

Toward the end, before I quit smoking, the cost of three packs a day was difficult to afford. The problem seemed not to turn on cutting the cost, as much as it did in allocating money for the cigarettes from some other (any other) budget item. Now, the less educated (and economically disadvantaged) seem to me to be the primary buyers; I think that a draconian tax on tobacco products might force many to break the habit. I support this strategy.

I have served as a mentor to seven people afflicted with lung cancer, five of whom died. If any smoker could watch a human being die in their arms from pulmonary insufficiency, I doubt that there is any way that they could continue smoking. Videos of this excruciating form of death would be a major selling point in smoking-cessation classes, which are entirely too bland. People think that death will come while they're sleeping, their head on a satin pillow, and a smile on their lips. Seeing someone slowly drown in their own body fluids will quickly change that perception, even those who may be heavily into denial.

The grief process entails many phases. The phrase that seems in my experience to last the longest is anger at the dead person for "willingly" disrupting the lives of survivors. "Why did he/she take himself away from me? He/she could have/should have quit smoking."

I am aggressively hostile toward restaurant management when they do not provide a nonsmoking area in their establishment, or when they don't enforce existing nonsmoking provisions. I also often carry a spray can containing DOG COLOGNE. This stuff smells like a hot July night in a whorehouse. Spraying it not only masks tobacco odor—it also clears the sinuses and brings a tear to the eye. Those who object are told that it is preferable to the stench of tobacco. The few who have reacted with threats of physical retaliation are quickly informed that I'm armed with pepper mace and a revolver, and if they still want to smoke, it would be a good plan to request a table out on the loading deck. End of discussion.

I Was Smoking Up to Three Packs a Day, Depending on My Level of Boredom—A Former Smoker

My eighteen-year history with nicotine began in 1973 at the age of fourteen. I remember that in 1973 not much was known about the harms of smoking cigarettes. Smoking was publicized as glamorous or cool. My circle of friends and I were typical, mildly rebellious teenagers. All of us had at least one parent who smoked. We stole cigarettes from our parents and dared each other to smoke them. When we started buying cigarettes at the local stores, no sales clerks ever refused to sell them to us. It would take us weeks to finish one pack. We continued at this pace until high school.

In high school, more serious cigarette smoking began: before school, lunchtime, after school, and evenings away from home. It was then that I think I became addicted. When I was forced to stay at home with my family, I used to climb out my bedroom window and sit on the roof and smoke.

I moved away to college immediately following high school, which meant I could smoke at any time, anywhere. At different times during college, I was smoking up to three packs a day depending on my level of boredom. After four to five years, the only pressure to quit smoking came from my parents, and upon graduation, I was employed with a company that accepted cigarette smoking.

Eleven years after graduation, the problems began; I had smoked for about sixteen to seventeen years. I started having difficult bouts with pleurisy and bronchitis, both of which recurred with increasing frequency. Now my family, friends, and doctor really pressured me to quit.

It seemed that in the public's eye, smokers were the scum of the earth. No-smoking policies were adopted everywhere, and I began seriously thinking about quitting. I didn't want to be seen as "scum of the earth" and I was concerned about my health. The turning point came when I visited a friend's father in hospital—he was dying of lung and bone cancer caused by cigarettes. I was horrified—he weighed 100 pounds or less and looked like he was already dead. He died two days after my visit.

I woke up the day after visiting him and decided that it would be the day I quit smoking: April 11. I smoked my last cigarette that morning at 7 and told myself to remember it, since it would be my last. I put all my cigarettes in the refrigerator and put on a nicotine patch. The only people I told that I had quit were my co-workers, and they didn't believe I would be successful. I continued with the patches, and after two weeks my boss decided that if I could quit, she could and did.

Every time I had the urge to smoke, I told myself that I was stronger than the cigarettes. I did not tell my family or friends about quitting until I had not smoked for one month. Within two weeks, I could breathe easier. I realized how bad cigarettes smell, which I could never do before. Eventually, I stopped the patches and began chewing Nicorette. I still chew Nicorette. I was able to make myself quit smoking, but I have not been able to convince others to quit.

I still feel that smokers are social outcasts, especially now with stricter regulations. I feel that all smokers are victims of the addictive power of cigarettes and are looked down upon by nonsmokers, most of whom have never been victims of this addiction.

My heart goes out to very addicted smokers. They do not know how they would feel if they didn't smoke. They know the harmful effects of smoking, but either do not acknowledge them or don't think anything will happen to them. I felt that cigarettes weren't harming me, then I quit. I've had numerous bladder disorders and surgeries, all of which I today feel cigarettes caused. Since I quit smoking, I have not had pleurisy or bronchitis.

Not Only Was He a Victim of Tobacco—So Were We—A Former Smoker

You could tell when he needed a cigarette: He became frustrated and short-tempered. It made us angry that he smoked, because he was not the only victim of his tobacco use, so were we!

Emotionally, it was difficult to have a smoker in the family. When my husband smoked, he did so in the garage. When he was done, the children would tease and scold him. He was sending them mixed messages: Do what I say, not what I do.

He participated in a well-known stop-smoking program and used the patch at different times. He would quit for less than six months. He tried changing brands, tried to save money in a jar—nothing worked. The children, relatives, and I were supportive, but all our efforts were unsuccessful until he was ready to quit for himself. You can't change another person's behavior.

I started smoking when I was sixteen. A friend encouraged me to try and I said, "Okay, why not?" When I wanted to have children, I decided to quit. I quit eighteen months before conception so that my body could clean itself out. That's when I learned how I was affected by nicotine and realized my addiction.

Breaking the smoking habit, especially when talking on the phone or driving, was tough.

Smokers Have a Hard Road to Travel—A Former Smoker

I am a laboratory and X-ray technician and scientist. I am also an emergency medical technician with our ambulance service. In my career, I have seen a lot of cancers and other illnesses caused by cigarettes.

I once had a girlfriend whose father had esophageal cancer. They told him it was from cigarette smoking. He died a long, slow, agonizing death. He just wasted away when he could no longer eat or hold the food down.

When I was twenty-one years old in college, one of my roommates gave me a cigarette because I was stressed over examinations and term papers. When I finally finished school and got my first job in a laboratory, I continued to smoke because it was hectic with hardly any time for breaks. Smoking helped. The only time I would stop and rest was when I had a cigarette, so I believed that it was relaxing. I enjoyed smoking. It is hard for nonsmokers to understand this, but it's true.

Three out of four people in the laboratory smoked. I smoked for ten years before I ever tried to quit. I tried to quit because of my mother. I made the decision to quit not for my sake but hers. It didn't work. All the physical and mental anguish you go through, you can't go through for somebody else. It has to be your decision to quit; you are the one that has to go through it.

I have tried to quit smoking three times unsuccessfully. I guess I wasn't really ready to quit—I enjoyed smoking too much. Finally, I decided to quit for myself. I went to a support group for smokers. The people were very honest. They told me that it would be difficult to quit, and that if I broke down and had a cigarette I should not let the guilt beat me down. They told me it was all right to have a cigarette if the feelings got too intense. I must have been ready to quit, because after that meeting I quit cold turkey.

I had a very hard time when I quit. I was physically sick for two weeks. Other people I have talked to who also quit did not have the physical sickness and the psychological and emotional turmoil that I did. I consider myself very lucky because the difficulty reinforced my determination to quit. I saw myself, knew I was hooked, and didn't like what I saw. The first five days without cigarettes were a breeze. Then I started to get headaches. Sick to my stomach. Chills. After that, the emotional upheaval took over. I would pick fights with my husband and drive him out of the house. Then I would feel guilty and cry for hours. I was a mess. That's when I knew for sure I had been hooked, and I decided I was never going to be hooked again. I knew I was never going to turn into that person again. Nothing I took was going to turn me into that person.

Quitting smoking is the hardest thing to do because it is an addiction—not only a physical addiction, but a psychological addiction. It has been over three years since I quit. Smokers have a hard road to travel.

You have to remember that smoking is legal. I don't believe anyone should be trying to stop others from smoking in their presence. If the room is well ventilated, there is no need to treat cigarette smokers as lepers. That's exactly the way we treat them. Now, they have passed legislation so that the only public place they can smoke is outside. I feel bad for them. Quitting smoking is hard enough, but then you have to deal with people harassing you. It's not right.

There Is Not One Cigarette That I Do Not Enjoy or Look Forward to—A Smoker Who Can't Quit

I taught myself how to smoke at fourteen; I "trained" on my father's Camel nonfilter cigarettes. I am now forty-two and smoke three packs of cigarettes a day.

I wanted to smoke to look "cool" like the other kids in my high school. I would come home from school and practice inhaling. Of course, I thought I would be able to throw them away long before I ever got hooked. Both of my parents were heavy smokers and so were my two older sisters. Currently, only one sister and I still smoke.

I smoked through three normal pregnancies knowing full well the possible damage to my children, but was still not able to quit. I knew all the medical, social, and financial consequences of smoking, so I don't believe that intelligence or lack of it has anything to do with the decision to keep smoking.

For the past twenty years, I have been waking every hour throughout the night for a cigarette. I smoke twenty-four hours a day and there is not one cigarette that I do not enjoy or look forward to. My family doctor tried to break my habit of waking up all night to smoke by giving me a prescription for seven sleeping pills. For seven nights, I slept through the entire night and it was very restful, but then on the eighth night I started waking up as usual. My doctor said that I was horribly "hooked" on nicotine and that I should just quit cold turkey.

I have tried three times unsuccessfully to quit. I have been to a couple of speakers on the subject and although everything made sense on a certain level, I couldn't wait to leave so that I could smoke. I tried the nicotine gum, cold turkey, and I have purchased the patch but have yet to try it. I have failed miserably at all my attempts to quit. I have tried cutting down to save money, and when that didn't work I went to rolling my own cigarettes, which I still do. My friends and family want me to quit, but I just can't yet.

My most recent and serious attempt to quit was about five years ago; it was just costing me too much money. I read books and truly thought I was ready to quit. But within twenty-four hours, I was vomiting, crying, and basically hysterical. I was a nervous wreck. I gave up and went to the store at 3 a.m. to purchase cigarettes.

Perhaps you might find this crazy, but 99.9% of the time I don't really want to quit. In Canada, the price of cigarettes alone should be enough of a deterrent, but obviously it is not enough of one for me.

As a single parent of three children, the money I spend could certainly go to better things, but I guess I think that cancer or any of the other smoking-related diseases won't happen to me. Although I don't believe that my family or myself have been in a crisis because of my smoking, I may not be the best judge of that.

I do have a cough, which I choose to ignore. And if I get a cold, it usually turns into pneumonia. I have seen my doctor for four bleeding ulcers, and he tells me that smoking aggravates the problem.

I have two sons and a daughter. Both my sons detest smoking and don't hesitate to let me know about it. My daughter is nineteen, and she began smoking at fourteen. I had hoped that she would be smarter than I was. I tried to tell her how incredible the addiction is, but to no avail. I certainly can't tell her what to do when I continue to smoke.

If I am invited somewhere that is "no smoking," I do not attend.

My personal wish is to see nicotine addiction treated as any other drug addiction. If we could be hospitalized or put in treatment centers paid for by workplace or other insurance, allowing us to take the time out of our lives to properly quit the way alcoholics are detoxified or heroin addicts helped through their withdrawal, the success rate would be far better. Certainly, it would be more helpful than simply harping at us to quit smoking. Increasing the price and banning smoking in certain places and all the other medical aids to date have just not worked.

I Consider Quitting to Be One of the Greatest Accomplishments of My Life—A Former Smoker

I quit smoking six years ago. My life had changed considerably; we had moved to Minneapolis in March and I quit smoking June 1. For the first time, I was in an environment that was hostile to smoking. The cost of cigarettes was outrageous and I immediately ran into people and places that didn't allow smoking. Georgia, where we lived before, was just the opposite—lots of smokers and cheap cigarettes. You could even smoke in the grocery store there! Maryland, where I lived and smoked for the seven years before Georgia, was mixed. I had friends who smoked. At the time, I had two good friends who tried to quit; one was successful and the other failed. I never thought of quitting, even though my father-in-law and mother-in-law both died during those years of tobacco-related illnesses.

I enjoyed smoking. Lots of people around me smoked. There was no negative feedback. (I avoided that by not smoking in front of my parents and relatives for years. They were religious.) Eventually, I did smoke in front of my parents. My mother now smokes about five cigarettes a day, but did not smoke when I was growing up or in college. My father quit smoking when he came home from WWII because he became very religious. I remember the men smoking in front of the church before services started, but not my dad.

I was starting to get restless in Georgia. My daughter was sixteen and I knew her best girlfriend smoked. My daughter was very rebellious and unhappy, and I was not setting a good example for her. I began to feel unintelligent—stupid and addicted. I cut down. I switched brands. I was miserable in the car with the children. Don't smoke here. Smoke there. Have fun. They're cheap.

Then I moved. I was doing the unpopular thing. I quit and am glad I did.

I was addicted to the entire concept of smoking, not just the nicotine. When I quit, I wore no patch and had few symptoms of nicotine withdrawal. I believe this is an individual matter. I miss all the motions and comforts of smoking, not the taste, smell, or nicotine effects. I did not go to a restaurant or bar for six weeks after I quit, and I still have trouble playing bridge without my cigarettes. Quitting is like losing your best friend. It changed my life.

Now, I drink very little and do not go bar hopping or just sit around and drink and chat with people. I have to be doing something, and I couldn't handle the alcohol without cigarettes—they just went together for me. I gained fifteen pounds over the first year before I changed my eating habits and started exercising regularly. Another lifestyle change! When I smoked, I kept my ideal weight with little thought; when others ate, I smoked. I miss that, but I adjusted my habits over time. It was not easy. I consider quitting to be one of the greatest accomplishments of my life. I expected that I would miss cigarettes forever and tried to take it one day at a time. I admitted to everyone that it was hard for me. I was patient with myself and accepted that it was hard work and, for the first several months, all consuming.

It's been six years and I still occasionally wish I could have a smoke, but I choose not to. I try not to push others, but I am very supportive of those who have quit or want to quit. There have been many, including my brother and his wife. They are very well educated, intelligent people, and it was a struggle, but they quit. My sister quit many times; she was a nicotine addict. She's been off the cigarettes for one and a half years and I still praise her and my brother.

My sister's house was in a constant state of tension for two years as she struggled to quit. Her husband and seven-year-old daughter put tremendous pressure on her. She smoked when they weren't around. She resented their pressure and hated herself for sneaking. She asked my advice as I had quit several years before. I said, "You'll quit when you quit."

My sixteen-year-old has no desire to be cool and smoke. She is a real purist about her body and I hope that continues. My husband was very supportive of the changes in our lives, but I know he still misses the partying that will be no more. It wasn't good for me and I couldn't handle it anymore. I had to accept myself with all my shortcomings.

CHAPTER 10

Conclusion—Beginning the Dialogue

In this final chapter, we will briefly summarize what the participants in our project told us about smoking in the USA; then we will offer some ideas on how people can move toward more openly and honestly communicating about smoking.

The effects of smoking on couple relationships can be devastating. For nonsmoking partners and those who have quit, issues of trust and intimacy are paramount. For smoking partners, feelings of guilt and shame are common if they believe their habit or addiction is harmful to their partners and other family members. These feelings are intensified by the pressure of other family members to quit, and disputes are common over issues of individual autonomy and over "the right to smoke." Physical intimacy can diminish among couples because of repulsion from the smell of smoke on the part of the nonsmoker, and diminished libido and impotence on the part of the smoker. "Why can't you quit when it is so damaging to you and to your loved ones?" And the answer is, "Because…"

Parent–child relationships can also be negatively affected by smoking. Parents feel humiliated and abused by the public, who may see smoking as evidence of bad parenting or even child abuse. Many parents feel guilt over harming their children's health or causing their children to take up smoking also. Many children of smokers told us about health problems related to smoking that they endured over the years, and how this damaged their relationships with their parents. Smoking parents who do not want their children to smoke express frustration that they cannot

I. Newman and J. DeFrain, *Tobacco Use and Intimate Relationships*,
https://doi.org/10.1007/978-3-319-92579-0_10

convince the younger generation that it is a mistake to take up smoking. Smoking children of nonsmoking parents sometimes hide their habit from parents for years.

Smokers who do not believe their smoking has adverse effects on their family almost always paint unflattering portraits of family members who are intolerant of their desire, need, and right to smoke. Smokers often express feelings of rejection and humiliation when asked not to smoke in their children's homes, around the grandchildren, or in their own homes when the extended family comes for a visit. Perhaps the most dramatic effects of smoking are seen on families dealing with the death of a loved one from smoking-related illness. Anger and feelings of guilt are common, and attempts often made to deal with the situation by imposing silence on the family and refusing to talk about the loss and why it happened. These struggles pull people further and further apart from each other.

Anger, silence, and secrecy are common in families of smokers. For the smoking parent, rejection of his smoking and denial of his right to smoke threatens his parental rights and authority, which makes him feel humiliated and hurt—like a child. The nonsmoking child's own fear for her parent's health as well as the health of her own family becomes reduced to an expansion of her authority as an adult and parent in her own right. Inevitably, these arguments veil the real emotions of insecurity, humiliation, and fear that both parent and adult child feel. These genuine feelings are masked by anger, silence, and ultimately, secrecy. The consequence of silence on occasions like these is the deliberate estrangement of family ties, unresolved and continued emotional pain. Certainly, these silences do not help the tobacco addict quit or the nonsmoker find ways to reconcile.

All the groups or people participating in the project—unrepentant smokers, smokers who wanted to quit but felt they couldn't, smokers who had quit, and lifelong smokers—included accounts of secrecy in their narratives, specifically that of "closet smoking." Smokers and nonsmokers alike believe that they have inviolable rights and many invoke the rhetoric of the Civil Rights Movement and American Independence in their narratives. Unrepentant smokers believe that nonsmokers are intolerant and hostile for no particular reason, that they are a privileged majority. Because smokers for the most part surround themselves with smokers rather than nonsmokers, and because the issue is often wrapped in deadening and tangible silence within families due to the tension surrounding it, many smokers do not believe that secondhand smoke poses a significant health risk to the nonsmoker.

For "born again" nonsmokers and lifelong nonsmokers, the effects of secondhand smoke are real and devastating. These populations together tend, for the most part, to see smokers as an indistinct, homogenous group of hostile, inconsiderate, and privileged people—a perspective that smokers also hold to be true of nonsmokers. For nonsmokers, especially those with severe respiratory ailments and other allergies, consistent exposure to smoke is a constant reminder of the power of smokers over their lives, health, and livelihood. No party around the issue of smoking can truly be said to have privilege, and the abuse of power only hurts all involved. Again, clearly what is missing is communication, understanding and support, and genuine civility.

Personal rights and the American way are commonly invoked in the battle over smoking. On both sides of the issue, smokers and non-smokers alike believe that they have inviolable, "God-given" rights. Unfortunately, like many American debates surrounding the contentious issues of choice, neither side of the issue appears to be able to listen to or understand the other.

So, is there a compromise to be found? It is clear from all of the narratives that hypocrisy on the part of the government is partially to blame. Nonsmokers would like the government to take a clear and resolute stance on tobacco use, and smokers for the most part feel that the government increasingly infringes on their civil rights while profiting from tobacco use. Furthermore, many smokers feel strongly that the anti-smoking movement is biased; after all, many products endanger the health of users and those surrounding them, such as alcohol or fatty foods. They believe that it is hypocritical of the government and mainstream society to restrict their rights, yet not treat alcoholism or obesity as equal issues. Obviously, this imbalance must be addressed; for the smoker, the discrimination and persecution is real.

Complex and contentious health issues swirl around the world of both the smoker and the nonsmoker. Many smokers, especially those who don't want to quit, feel like they are the healthiest people they know, and justify their self-diagnoses, attributing any health problems, if they exist, to age. It is impossible for smokers who deny the effects of tobacco use on their own health to acknowledge the effects of secondhand smoke to nonsmokers. Some smokers are very aware of the effects of second-hand smoke and feel guilty about their addictions, but helpless when confronted with the difficulties of quitting. For these smokers, quitting is still a challenge, and fear for their health and the health of loved ones must compete with fear of going without tobacco. Unfortunately, because of the tenacity of addiction, many of these smokers do not quit until their worst fears are realized and they are confronted with a diagnosis of cancer or another smoke-related disease. For those that do quit, a few resume smoking because of weight gain, a fate apparently worse than smoke-related disease and death.

Nonsmokers and former smokers who suffer from allergies due to exposure to secondhand smoke describe in detail the history of their problems with tobacco, leaving no room for doubt that secondhand smoke constitutes a constant and eminent risk to their lives in a myriad of ways. Many have been subjected to secondhand smoke from childhood and recall the oppressive atmospheres they grew up in as directly responsible for chronic health problems that began when they were children.

Smokers and nonsmokers alike generally feel that the medical establishment treats the issue of tobacco use ineffectively, inappropriately, and inhumanely. Smokers feel that doctors, nurses, and medical facilities fail to take into account the needs of smokers as addicts; many feel that such treatment is discriminating. Smokers and nonsmokers express the need for medical institutions to treat patients who smoke as people with addictions, rather than weak-willed/minded tobacco abusers. Unfortunately, many smokers write of avoiding health checkups and care because of constant harassment, denial of care, and other "abuse" from doctors and nurses, a fact that may delay the decision to quit and the early detection and timely treatment of disease.

Tobacco has an enormous amount of power in the lives of both smokers and nonsmokers. For both groups of people, tobacco can determine one's daily activities, livelihood, relationships, and health. Tobacco use and nonuse can determine if a person lives or dies, keeps or loses a job, falls in love with or is repelled by a potential partner, remains married or divorces. If one is allergic or addicted, the entire day's routine, indeed, one's whole life must take into account this fact—a chronic smoker cannot leave the house without his cigarettes and lighter and can only go where he will be able to smoke; a nonsmoker with severe allergies must also plan her daily activities to avoid exposure to smoke and other irritants.

Control is a central issue here for many smokers and nonsmokers. Nonsmokers, particularly those with severe allergies and other respiratory problems, often feel like smokers deprive them of control over their lives, livelihood, and health. Many smokers also feel that they have lost their autonomy, admitting that the addiction to tobacco rules their lives. Tobacco becomes part of their lifestyle; smokers who attempt to quit have a difficult time adjusting to a routine without a cigarette in hand because the rituals of smoking become part of every minute of one's day. What initially seems to be an enjoyable accessory to the routines of daily life inevitably becomes necessary—the cigarette becomes central.

Many relationships have been constructed or destroyed around tobacco. Smokers and nonsmokers tend to avoid striking up or maintaining friendships or acquaintances with each other. Both sides admit a sense of social ostracism because of their relationship to tobacco—smokers feel they are targets of discrimination and abuse, and militant nonsmokers feel that because of their "extreme" positions on tobacco, they too are isolated and silenced. Because many smokers and nonsmokers avoid each other in social and other situations, both groups cultivate stereotypes of each other.

In spite of all the negative consequences of smoking, people still begin and continue the habit for a variety of social, psychological, and cultural reasons. While most recall smoking their first cigarette as youth, especially in adolescence, some do pick up the habit much later in life. Of those that begin in youth and young adulthood, many smokers report growing up around role models who smoked, including parents and other close relatives, teachers, coaches, heads of churches, movie stars, as well as peers. These youth choose to smoke in imitation of role models because they simply want to be like the adults or peers they admire and to feel connected to the group, to raise self-esteem, or to be rebellious, sophisticated, glamorous, mysterious. Those who pick up the habit later in life also do so for a variety of reasons; some report smoking to control their weight, to emulate another who smokes, and even to self-medicate on the advice of other smokers.

Why smokers continue to light up and inhale is much simpler—addiction, stressful lives, and pure pleasure. Many smokers hold to the belief that smoking is a cure for various ailments, particularly stress and anxiety. Cigarettes are like a close companion and friend, present through all the trials of life and therefore difficult, sometimes impossible, to let go.

Others wax poetic about the sensuality of smoking, and love everything about the cigarette—its smell, the smoke, the physical ritual of smoking.

Although quite a few smokers deny that they might be addicted to tobacco, claiming they can quit if they want to, the majority of former smokers and many who have attempted to quit are quick to admit addiction. Many only realize they are addicted when they attempt to quit. Quitting smoking entails physical and mental anguish: smokers face withdrawal symptoms from nervousness to headaches, and constantly crave the release that can only come from a cigarette. Because quitting is so difficult, the process is usually a trial for everyone involved, particularly loved ones.

The physical act of smoking (described as sensual by many) as much as the chemical effects of tobacco make quitting next to impossible for the majority of smokers. Cigarettes become an integral part of a daily routine. Lifestyle changes are necessary in order to reduce or quit smoking, something not very many of us have the discipline and will to enact.

Smokers attempt to quit for a variety of reasons. Those reasons can determine the success or failure of their efforts; for example, to quit because a loved one pressures you to quit leads most often to secret smoking and resentment. Rarely is a smoker able to quit unless he or she genuinely wants to. Smokers who do want to quit are generally concerned about their health as well as the health of those around them. Unfortunately, many only quit for good when their health is in critical condition—after having being diagnosed with cancer and prior to radical treatment such as surgery.

The methods for quitting are numerous and costly: the patch, gum, stop-smoking programs, counseling, hypnosis, and acupuncture. Most former smokers report that the most successful method is going "cold turkey." Some smokers are able to do just that; others must first reduce the number and frequency of cigarettes before quitting altogether. Early in the process of attempting to quit, the realities of smoking as an addiction begin to set in, and the illusions of many that they are in control inevitably fall to pieces. Such an experience can be traumatic and eventually freeing. While some former smokers still crave cigarettes, missing the sensations of smoking as well as its rituals, many learn to hate everything about smoking and cannot even imagine how they started in the first place. Some even become active in the anti-smoking movement—"born-again nonsmokers."

What, Then, Can Be Done?

The battle over smoking in this country has raged for many years on television, on the radio, in newspapers and magazines, on the Internet; and, it seems to be spreading around the world before our eyes. When we began this project several years ago, we wanted to step back away from the headlines and the noise of the controversy and go deep into the personal lives of those most affected by smoking.

And that is precisely what has happened. We asked for volunteers, for people whose lives had been touched in some way by smoking. A simple, basic question drove the project: "How has smoking affected your life?"

The volunteers in our study told us many stories: happy stories, playful stories, angry stories, sad stories. They told of their love affair with cigarettes; they told of their hatred for the vice and its purveyors. Their emotions ran the gamut of human emotion, and their opinions came in from every conceivable angle in the discussion of smoking in American life. There was no consensus. There was no agreement. There was no compromise. There was no solution to the dilemma of smoking in American life.

But, if there is to be a solution, it will come, as always, from positive communication among all those affected by smoking, and that really is every one of us. Currently, we are divided into two basic camps, or tribes, if you will. The smoking and nonsmoking camps can be broken down into sub-groups adding further complexity to the situation. If we are to make any progress in the shrill and continuing dialogue over smoking, the volume will have to be turned down and we will have to shed the mantle of self-righteousness and listen with our hearts to each other. This is not a battle between the forces of good and the forces of evil. This often is a battle between people who dearly love each other and, for the life of them, can find no common ground for the beginnings of constructive dialogue, having experienced the problems of addiction as both smokers and nonsmokers. For both smokers and nonsmokers to take back control of their lifestyles, dialogue is essential.

About the Authors

Ian Newman sneaked cigarettes as a youngster in New Zealand from his older sister's boyfriends and his own friends. His father smoked and his mother smoked occasionally and reluctantly after dinners with friends. He remembers the wife of one of his dad's best friends, a couple who often joined his family for dinner, always blowing beautiful smoke rings. It was as if she was an artist with smoke. At the time, none of this was out of the ordinary. In retrospect, he now makes the connection between the smoke rings and the fact that she was dead of inoperable cancer 10 years later.

When he was as tall as the top button on his dad's waistcoat his dad quit smoking. Ian never knew why. In the 1950s, it is unlikely it was due to published reports on the dangers to health.

While a doctoral student at the University of Illinois in the late 1960s, Ian was a research assistant for the antismoking education study at the University of Illinois, led by his professor, William Creswell Jr. This was one of the earliest research studies sponsored by the US Government to study adolescent smoking behaviors, in light of the findings published in 1964 in the first Surgeon General's Report on Smoking and Health.

As a student in health education and anthropology, a believer in the value of participant-observer research, he decided he should experience firsthand the feeling of smoking. Success was tracked with a large jar that slowly filled with cigarette butts. He likes to recall how he failed to become a smoker but succeeded in gaining some insight into the process.

I. Newman and J. DeFrain, *Tobacco Use and Intimate Relationships*,
https://doi.org/10.1007/978-3-319-92579-0

Leaving Illinois with a new Ph.D. and a wife (Enid from Trinidad) and son, Ian went to the University of Tennessee. The excitement of participant observation and interest in health-related behavior led to long excursions into the back roads of the Cumberland Mountains to learn from backcountry folk about their health and their lifestyles, to sample their moonshine, and to discuss the "evils" imposed by the coal companies. They weren't always welcoming of strangers but, once started, they enjoyed the opportunity to talk and reminisce. Occasionally, he took along his 4-year-old son as a ticket to hospitality.

After postdoctoral study at Harvard University School of Public Health with Professors Marjori Young and Jeanette Simmons, Ian moved his family to New Delhi to the South East Regional Office of the World Health Organization. His supervisor and mentor was Dr. V. S. Ramakrishna, a Brahman Hindu, trained as a surgeon, who elected to work in public health and had a distinguished career in the Indian public health service before joining WHO. He and Ian shared a passion to see the world through other people's eyes. Life in India and work in Thailand, Nepal, and Sri Lanka reinforced this curiosity. Then, it was back to the USA where the children, 3 sons, could experience an American education and Ian could pursue his interest in the connection between behavior and health.

The study of tobacco use, an area of study in which only a few scientists were working in the 1960s, had engaged the interest and curiosity of social scientists, public health workers, and disease prevention organizations. Population survey and medical data on tobacco use and its effects accumulated, but few studies considered the realities of individuals affected by tobacco.

Over the years, Ian's interest has gravitated to understanding adolescent alcohol use and then adolescent alcohol use in China. He considers alcohol use an even more interesting behavior than tobacco use, because, unlike tobacco, a little alcohol use seems to have health benefits. From a public health perspective, we would be better off without both tobacco and alcohol, but that will not happen; so the challenge is to reduce the risks of irresponsible use and to find ways to reduce chances of harm when use does occur. For the last 25 years, he has been teaching in, traveling through, and learning about China. He initiated and led a 10-year program of annual workshops for health education workers in Inner Mongolia. His research on adolescent alcohol use has led to the development and refinement of a Chinese adolescent alcohol expectancy scale, the Chinese adolescent alcohol self-efficacy scale, and a Chinese adolescent cultural orientation scale. For the past 10 years, he has spent time in small villages and towns in rural China talking to alcohol makers about their craft, it's heritage, and how and why alcohol is integrated into daily life without significant problems. He provided public health expertise to the University of Nebraska's successful initiative to reduce binge drinking by college students, and he has led a consortium of Nebraska colleges and universities in efforts to reduce drinking and drunk driving among their students. He has published more than 150 research papers and given almost 300 presentations and keynote addresses at national and international meetings. A textbook, *School Health Practice*, authored by Ian and his professor Bill Creswell, completed 10 editions.

John DeFrain's father one evening back in the 1950s got out a cup of coffee, a bottle of whiskey, and a pack of cigarettes. John was, perhaps, 12 years old at the time. His father at that stage of life was a coffee drinker, drank alcohol rarely, and smoked on occasion. "Try some of this coffee," he urged his son. John took a big swig of coffee, choked and coughed, but managed to get it down. His dad then urged him to drink a shot of whiskey, straight down. More choking, coughing, some sputtering. This experiment was followed up with a long drag on a cigarette, and the result was similar though the additive effects of all three experiments made the experience even more unpleasant: choking, coughing, sputtering, and perhaps a bit of gagging as well.

Dad died of prostate cancer before John ever got a chance to ask him what the purpose of these experiments really was. Dad was a professional in public health for 37 years. Perhaps he wanted John to stay away from coffee, alcohol, and cigarettes. Or maybe he wanted to introduce them to me in our home, up front, rather than me sneaking out to experiment on my own with friends. Maybe he just wanted a good laugh. John will never know.

But the fact of the matter is, John has never drunk a cup of coffee. The glass of wine he has, say, once a year to be social just makes him sleepy. And he never has smoked another cigarette, though he tried marijuana in the 1960s and concluded it was just an exotic and illegal-type of cigarette that made you choke, cough, and sputter. Because of his allergic response to smoke, John's throat constricts severely when he tries to smoke, and being around smoke gives him a severe headache and congested lungs.

Would John recommend such an approach to parents who hope to condition their children against coffee, alcohol, cigarettes, or whatever? Not necessarily. He knows alcoholics who were given beer as babies to quiet them down, so what turned out to be aversive stimuli for John became a comfort for other youngsters.

John met his lifelong partner Nikki DeFrain when they were both 15 years old. When people ask why neither smokes nor drinks, she tends to reply that her father was an alcoholic and she associates alcohol with too many bad memories. "Besides," she continues, "in high school when all our friends were out smoking and drinking, John and I were always alone together enjoying the more alluring pleasures of young love."

John is a professor emeritus in the Department of Child, Youth and Family Studies at the University of Nebraska-Lincoln. His research interests over the past 40 years have focused on how to help people create strong, happy, and healthy families. He was drawn to the idea of writing a book on smoking, because so little is known on how it effects our personal lives—our intimate lives behind closed doors with our loved ones. His other recent books include *Marriages and Families: Intimacy, Diversity, and Strengths* (*9th ed.*); *Strong Families Around the World: Strengths-Based Research and Perspectives*; *Family Violence from a Global Perspective*; *Surviving and Transcending a Traumatic Childhood: The Dark Thread*; *The World of Bereavement: Cultural Perspectives on Death in Families*; and *The Chinese Family Today*. Working on this book has made John much more sensitive to the difficult personal dilemmas people face in life surrounding smoking, and especially sensitive to the challenges smokers face. His disdain for Big Tobacco is, however, undiminished.

Appendix A: Why and How We Did This Study

Since 1964, when the US Surgeon General issued the first report on smoking and health,[1] there has been an enormous accumulation of data about the medical and economic consequences of cigarette smoking. A staggering 480,000 people age 35 and older die each year from smoking-related diseases, a number which includes 41,000 people who die from secondhand smoke—that is, smoke from other people's cigarettes.[2] If American young people continue to smoke at their present rate, we can expect 5.6 million of them to die prematurely from smoking-related diseases, about one of every 13 Americans age 17 or younger alive today.[2]

The total annual economic cost of cigarette smoking exceeds $300 billion: $170 billion from direct medical care expenses and $156 billion from lost productivity due to premature death and exposure to secondhand smoke.[2,3]

The smoking debate is fueled by statistics like this. Efforts to reduce the impact of smoking in terms of disease and costs have included restricting places where smoking is allowed, encouraging nonsmokers to assert their rights to smoke-free air, and dramatically increasing cigarette prices through taxation.

In all the ongoing debate, there is rarely any discussion about what is happening in the living rooms, kitchens, front porches of tobacco users and their families.

There is still a fixation on statistical data. Statistics serve a purpose; they describe groups well, but not individuals. Statistics are impersonal;

I. Newman and J. DeFrain, *Tobacco Use and Intimate Relationships*,
https://doi.org/10.1007/978-3-319-92579-0

they provide logic and rationality to the debate, but not the emotional side of the story. We see a number—like 480,000—and our eyes glaze over. That's a large number. It's impersonal. We have little recognition that the 480,000 are individual people—smokers and their loved ones—each with a story to tell. Each 1 of the 480,000 is a father, a mother, a husband, a wife, a sister, a brother, a friend, and a lover. How that person got to be a part of the statistic is a story that cannot be imparted by the statistic.

We understand and respect statistical data and appreciate the elegance of the messages it conveys; but we wanted to know more about the people whose stories are hidden within the statistics that describe smoking rates, medical conditions, and other costs of smoking. We wanted to meet the smokers and the people who are affected by smokers' stories.

Pilot Study

One of the authors, John DeFrain, had successfully used media postings to recruit volunteers to share personal experiences about such topics as family strengths and challenges, sudden infant death, stillbirth, single parenthood, and so forth. It seemed that this same strategy might gain us access and insight to the experiences of smokers and those affected by smokers' behavior.

So, we sent letters to 67 newspapers selected from the *Gale Directory of Publications & Broadcast Media*, to the newspaper editor, explaining the project. An unknown number of newspapers published our plea for volunteers who were willing to fill out an anonymous, confidential 10-page questionnaire asking about their tobacco stories.

Twelve volunteers wrote to ask for the questionnaire. We mailed them each a questionnaire and received 9 completed questionnaires. Based on the results of this pilot test, we rewrote the questionnaire with more specific questions to encourage stories of consequences of tobacco use on members of the family and family relationships.

First Phase

We then mailed press releases to 494 newspapers (not used in the pilot study) selected from the *Gale Directory*. In addition, we placed a notice of the study in *AARP Bulletin*, *Modern Maturity*, *Americans for Nonsmokers Rights Update*, and *Smoking and Health Review*.

We received replies mainly from people we considered "survivors"—people who had a loved one sicken or die from tobacco-related disease.

Second Phase

We wanted to hear more stories from smokers so we wrote two ***different*** press releases, one seeking cooperation from smokers and one from survivors. We selected 325 additional newspapers from the *Gale Directory* (not used in either the pilot study or the first phase). We first placed the addressed envelopes into zip-code order. Then, we placed every other envelope into one of 2 piles. One hundred twelve newspapers got the press release seeking survivors; 113 newspapers got the press release seeking smokers. We kept a record of which city received which press release. We checked that no city got both versions of the press release. When volunteers responded, we sent the Smoker's questionnaire or the Survivor's questionnaire, based on which city/newspaper they responded from.

Questionnaires

For the second phase, we created the Smoker's Questionnaire (Appendix B) and the Survivor's Questionnaire (Appendix C).

Third Phase

Next, we placed our request for smokers' stories in the newsletters of the American Smokers Alliance, the Smokers' Rights Alliance, Inc., and Californians Against Restrictive Legislation. We placed our request for survivors' stories in the newsletters of Group Against Smoker's Pollution (GASP), Doctors Ought to Care (DOC), and Americans for Non-Smokers Rights.

Over the course of all phases of the study, a total of 225 people wrote to us to request questionnaires, and 139 people returned a completed questionnaire. The replies ranged from terse (one- or two-word answers to our questions) to eloquent—some writers sending in many typed or hand-written pages describing their experience in profound detail.

We read and reread the completed questionnaires. Practically, all were anonymous but some individuals sought special replies about specific questions. Replies were sent but the questionnaires remained anonymous. In some cases, individuals, mostly smokers, added comments impugning our motives but nevertheless providing wonderful insights and seemed genuinely interested that somebody had bothered to ask about their opinions and experiences.

It is the words of these smokers and their family members that provided the themes that shaped this book.

Sources

1. U.S. Department of Health, Education and Welfare (January 1964). Smoking and Health: Report of the Advisory Committee to the Surgeon General Public Health Service. Washington, DC: U.S. Department of Health, Education and Welfare, Public Health Service, CDC, Report No. 1103.
2. U.S. Department of Health and Human Services. The Health Consequences of Smoking—50 Years of Progress. A Report of the Surgeon General. Atlanta: U.S. Department of Health and Human Services, Centers for Disease Control and Prevention, National Center for Chronic Disease Prevention and Health Promotion, Office on Smoking and Health, 2014 (accessed June 15, 2017).
3. Xu, X., Bishop, E. E., Kennedy, S. M., Simpson, S. A., & Pechacek, T. F. (2015). Annual healthcare spending attributable to cigarette smoking: An update. *American Journal of Preventive Medicine*, *48*(3), 326–333.

Appendix B: The Questionnaire for Smokers

The Social and Psychological Impact of Tobacco Use: How Tobacco Affects Our Lives

This questionnaire has two parts.

The *first part* is for you to tell us your personal story about what it is like to be a smoker or a chewer in today's society. We want you to tell us about the things that happen to you because you use tobacco, the way you are treated, how you feel, how you respond, and what you tell other people. Does your tobacco use affect your relations with your family, your employer, or your friends? Does tobacco use affect your future?

Don't worry about spelling, punctuation, or correct word usage. Simply tell us your story or stories. These are important to us. Include all the details. Add extra sheets to the survey if you need to.

The *second part* of this questionnaire, which begins on page 208, is a series of questions about specific experiences related to tobacco use.

Please complete both parts of the questionnaire and return it to us in the postage-paid envelope we have provided.

If you know others who may be interested in helping us by sharing their experiences, please suggest them to contact us by mail or phone for a questionnaire.

We have a separate questionnaire for people who have had a loved one sick or die from smoking or chewing tobacco. If you know of a person who would like to share their thoughts on what happened in their family

I. Newman and J. DeFrain, *Tobacco Use and Intimate Relationships*,
https://doi.org/10.1007/978-3-319-92579-0

because of tobacco, please tell them about our study and ask them to contact us.

Thank you for your help.

Part One:

Tell us what it's like to be a tobacco-user in today's society.

We want as much information and detail as possible. Add extra pages if you want to, or write on the backs of these pages if you need more space.

In the original survey, there were four blank 8 1/2 X 11 pages provided after the Part One question, with a note to encourage people to add more pages and to write as much as they needed.

Part Two:

Now we want to ask you some specific questions about your experience.

The Part Two questions are all listed here. The original survey left space after the open-ended questions for 1-2 paragraph written responses, and gave writers permission to write on the back of the paper and add more pages as needed.

1. Do people ever ask you not to smoke or chew in their presence?

   Yes ____
   No ____

   How does this make you feel?

   What do you usually do?

   What would you like to do?

2. How do you feel about regulations restricting smoking to certain locations?

3. Raising taxes on tobacco products is sometimes suggested as a way to discourage tobacco use. How do you react to this suggestion?

4. Have you ever violated a nonsmoking ordinance?

   Yes ____
   No ____

   How did it make you feel?

5. Have your children ever talked to you about your tobacco use?

   Yes ____
   No ____

   What did they say?

   How did it make you feel?

6. What do you think about tobacco advertising?

7. What attracts you to the brand you smoke or chew?

8. What is the attitude of your spouse or best friend to your tobacco use?

   If they are not happy about your smoking or chewing, have you tried to do anything about it?

9. Do you agree with the restrictions on the sale of tobacco products to young people?

   Yes ____
   No ____
   Please explain.

10. Have you ever been involved in actions to repeal restrictions on tobacco use?

   Yes ____
   No ____

   What were the restrictions and what did you do?

11. What is the most pleasurable thing about tobacco use?

12. If you ever had difficulty dealing with a tobacco-related situation, did you turn to someone for help?

   Yes ____
   No ____

   If yes, who did you turn to and what did you want them to do to help?

Before you go on, we need answers to a few questions about you.

13. Gender

   Female ____
   Male ____

14. Age: ____ years

15. Residence

   In a town or a city ____
   On a farm ____
   Not on a farm, but outside of a town or city ____

16. Employment

    Student ____
    Employed ____
    Unemployed ____
    Retired ____

17. Please describe your job. ______________________________

18. Marital status:

    Single, never married ____
    Married ____
    Divorced ____
    Widow/Widower ____

19. Education

    High school or less ____
    College degree or some college ____
    Graduate/professional school ____

20. Have any of your close friends or relatives died of any tobacco-related diseases?

    Yes ____
    No ____
    If yes, please explain.

21. Describe your smoking.

    I don't smoke and never did. ____
    I experimented a few times but never smoked as many as 100 cigarettes. ____
    I was a regular smoker for ____ years but quit ____ years ago. ____
    I smoke now and have done so for ____ years. ____

22. How would you describe your smoking today?
    - I don't smoke. ____
    - I am an occasional smoker and smoke about ____ cigarettes per day. ____
    - I am a regular smoker and smoke about ____ cigarettes per day. ____
    - (1 pack = 20 cigarettes)

23. Describe your use of chewing tobacco and/or snuff.
    - I don't chew or use snuff and never did. ____
    - I experimented a few times but never chewed or used snuff regularly. ____
    - I was a regular user for ____ years but quit ____ years ago. ____
    - I chew or use snuff and have done so for ____ years. ____

24. If you chew or use snuff now, how would you describe your use?
    - I don't chew or use snuff. ____
    - I am an occasional user. About ____ chews a day. ____
    - I am a regular user. About ____ chews a day. ____

25. If you chew or use snuff now, are you trying to quit or reduce your use?
    - Yes ____
    - No ____
    - Please explain.

26. If you have ever used tobacco, tell us how you first began, how old you were, what were the circumstances, and who else was involved.

27. After you began to use tobacco what encouraged you to continue using it?

28. If you ever tried to quit or reduce the amount of tobacco you used, when did you try? Why did you try to quit/reduce? What happened?

29. What was/is the most difficult part of quitting or reducing tobacco use?

30. Do you think you are (or were) addicted to tobacco? How do (did) you know? If you consider yourself addicted, please tell us what the addiction is like.

Appendix C: The Questionnaire for Survivors

The Social and Psychological Impact of Tobacco Use: How Tobacco Affects Our Lives

This questionnaire has two parts.

The *first part* is for you to tell us your personal story of what it is like to have a loved one sick or die from smoking or chewing tobacco. We want you to tell us about the things that happened to you and your family because of the smoking- or chewing-related illness or death. How did you feel? How did you cope? How did it affect your family, your relationships with other people, your attitudes, hopes, and dreams?

Don't worry about spelling, punctuation, or correct word usage. Simply tell us why and how tobacco affected you, who else was involved, over what period of time, how the story began, and if and how it was ever resolved. These are all important to us. (Add extra sheets if you wish to include more details.) We simply are trying to get a better understanding of how tobacco use really affects families and individuals.

The *second part* of this questionnaire, which begins on page 217, is a series of questions asking you about some specific experiences related to tobacco use.

Please complete both parts of the questionnaire and return it to us in the postage-paid envelope we have provided.

If you know others who may be interested in helping us by sharing their experiences, please suggest them to contact us by mail or phone for a questionnaire.

I. Newman and J. DeFrain, *Tobacco Use and Intimate Relationships*,
https://doi.org/10.1007/978-3-319-92579-0

We have a separate questionnaire for people who are tobacco users. If you know of a person who would like to share their thoughts on what it is like to be a smoker or chewer in today's society, please tell them about our study and ask them to contact us.

Thank you for your help.

Part One:

Tell us what it was like to have a loved one get sick or die from smoking or chewing tobacco.

We want as much information and detail as possible. Add extra pages if you want to, or write on the backs of these pages if you need more space.

In the original survey, there were four blank 8 1/2 X 11 pages provided after the Part One question, with a note to encourage people to add more pages and to write as much as they needed.

Part Two:

Now we want to ask you some specific questions about your experience.

The Part Two questions are all listed here. The original survey left space after the open-ended questions for 1-2 paragraph written responses, and gave writers permission to write on the back of the paper and add more pages as needed

1. What is the hardest part of watching someone who is sick or dying from tobacco use?

2. Did you ever try to get someone (could be yourself) to quit or reduce their use of tobacco?

Yes	____	If yes, who?	
No	____	Self	____
		Spouse	____
		Child	____
		Parent	____
		Grandparent	____
		Close friend	____
		Other relative	____
		Other	____ (please explain)

How did it go?

3. Did you ever try to get someone (could be yourself) to go to a quit-smoking or a quit-chewing program?

    Yes ____
    No ____
    Please explain

4. Did you ever try to get a woman (could be yourself) to stop tobacco use because she was pregnant? OR try to get a man (could be yourself) to stop because his spouse was expecting?

    Yes ____
    No ____
    If yes, what happened?

5. Did you ever try to get someone (could be yourself) to not spend so much money on smoking or chewing?

    Yes ____
    No ____
    If yes, how did they react?

6. Did you ever try to get someone to do something about someone else's smoking?

    Yes ____
    No ____
    Please explain.

7. Did you ever try to get someone (could be yourself) to see a doctor for a condition that might be related to smoking or chewing?

    Yes ____
    No ____
    If yes, how did it go?

8. Did you ever try to get someone (could be yourself) to take their medication for a condition caused by tobacco use?
   Yes ____
   No ____
   If yes, did they accept your suggestion?

9. Did you ever try to help someone dying of a tobacco caused illness?
   Yes ____
   No ____
   If yes, what did they do and how did you feel about it?

10. Did you ever try to help a friend or relative who was grieving because of the loss of someone to a tobacco-related death?
    Yes ____
    No ____
    Please explain.

11. Did you ever try to get someone to not smoke in your presence?
    Yes ____
    No ____
    What happened?

12. Did you ever try to get someone (could be yourself) to not smoke around children?
    Yes ____
    No ____
    What happened?

13. Did you ever try to convince someone not to start using tobacco?
    Yes ____
    No ____
    Please explain.

14. Have you ever been involved in educational, policy, or political activities to discourage or prohibit tobacco use?
    Yes ____
    No ____
    What happened?

15. Did you ever try to get your employer to provide a tobacco-free work environment?
    Yes ____
    No ____
    What was your employer's reaction?

16. Did you ever try to get someone (could be yourself) to enforce smoke-free or tobacco-free regulations?
    Yes ____
    No ____
    Please explain.

17. Did you ever try to limit or stop anti-tobacco efforts at your home or at your work place?
    Yes ____
    No ____
    Please explain.

18. When you were having difficulty dealing with a tobacco-related situation, did you turn to someone for help?
    Yes ____
    No ____
    If yes, did it help? How did it help?

19. When you were trying to get someone to change their tobacco use did other people (close to you) support or hinder your efforts?
    Yes ____
    No ____
    Please explain.

20. What do you think about the way tobacco products are advertised?

Before you go on, we need answers to a few questions about you.

21. Gender
    - Female ____
    - Male ____

22. Age: ____ years

23. Residence
    - In a town or a city ____
    - On a farm ____
    - Not on a farm, but outside of a town or city ____

24. Employment
    - Student ____
    - Employed ____
    - Unemployed ____
    - Retired ____

25. Please describe your job. ________________________________

26. Marital status:
    - Single, never married ____
    - Married ____
    - Divorced ____
    - Widow/Widower ____

27. Education
    High school or less ____
    College degree or some college ____
    Graduate/professional school ____

28. Have any of your close friends or relatives of friends died of tobacco-related diseases?
    Yes ____
    No ____
    What was their relationship to you?

29. Have you ever seen tobacco use cause problems in a family?
    Yes ____
    No ____
    What happened?

If you have ever used, smoked, or chewed tobacco, please answer the following questions.

30. Describe your smoking.
    I don't smoke and never did. ____
    I experimented a few times but never smoked as many as 100 cigarettes. ____
    I was a regular smoker for ____ years but quit ____ years ago. ____
    I smoke now and have done so for ____ years. ____

31. How would you describe your smoking today?
    I don't smoke. ____
    I am an occasional smoker and smoke

about ____ cigarettes per day. ____
I am a regular smoker and smoke about ____ cigarettes per day. ____
(1 pack = 20 cigarettes)

32. Describe your use of chewing tobacco and/or snuff.
I don't chew or use snuff and never did. ____
I experimented a few times but never chewed or used snuff regularly. ____
I was a regular user for ____ years but quit ____ years ago. ____
I chew or use snuff and have done so for ____ years. ____

33. If you chew or use snuff now, how would you describe your use?
I don't chew or use snuff. ____
I am an occasional user. About ____ chews a day. ____
I am a regular user. About ____ chews a day. ____

34. If you chew or use snuff now, are you trying to quit or reduce your use?
Yes ____
No ____
How is it going? What's the hardest part?

35. If you have ever used tobacco, tell us how you first began, how old you were, what were the circumstances, and who else was involved.

36. After you began to use tobacco what made you continue to use tobacco?

37. When was the first time you tried to quit or reduce the amount of tobacco you used? Why did you try to quit/reduce? What happened?

38. What was/is the most difficult part of quitting or reducing tobacco use?

39. When and how did you realize you were addicted to tobacco?

Bibliography

Apelberg, B. J., Hepp, L. M., Avila-Tang, E., Gundel, L., Hammond, S. K., Hovell, M. F., et al. (2013). Environmental monitoring of secondhand smoke exposure. *Tobacco Control, 22*(3), 147–155. https://doi.org/10.1136/tobaccocontrol-2011-050301.

Avila-Tang, E., Al-Delaimy, W. K., Ashley, D. L., Benowitz, N., Bernert, J. T., Kim, S., et al. (2013). Assessing secondhand smoke using biological markers. *Tobacco Control, 22*(3), 164–171. https://doi.org/10.1136/tobaccocontrol-2011-050298.

BinDhim, N. F., Freeman, B., & Trevena, L. (2014). Pro-smoking apps for smartphones: The latest vehicle for the tobacco industry? *Tobacco Control, 23*(1), e4-2012-050598. Epub October 22, 2012. https://doi.org/10.1136/tobaccocontrol-2012-050598.

Brandt, A. M. (2009). *The cigarette century: The rise, fall, and deadly persistence of the product that defined America*. New York: Basic Books.

Bullen, C., Howe, C., Laugesen, M., McRobbie, H., Parag, V., Williman, J., & Walker, N. (2013). Electronic cigarettes for smoking cessation: A randomised controlled trial. *The Lancet, 382*(9905), 1629–1637. https://doi.org/10.1016/s0140-6736(13)61842-5.

Burns, E. (2007). *The smoke of the gods: A social history of tobacco*. Philadelphia: Temple University Press.

Cahill, K., & Lancaster, T. (2014). Workplace interventions for smoking cessation. *Cochrane Database of Systematic Reviews*, (2). https://doi.org/10.1002/14651858.cd003440.pub4.

Centers for Disease Control, National Center for Chronic Disease Prevention and Health Promotion, Office on Smoking and Health. (2016). *Tobacco-Related Mortality* (Fast Facts and Fact Sheets). Available from https://www.

I. Newman and J. DeFrain, *Tobacco Use and Intimate Relationships*, https://doi.org/10.1007/978-3-319-92579-0

cdc.gov/tobacco/data_statistics/fact_sheets/health_effects/tobacco_related_mortality/index.htm.

Centers for Disease Control, National Center for Chronic Disease Prevention and Health Promotion, Office on Smoking and Health. (2017a). *Economic Trends in Tobacco* (Fast Facts and Fact Sheets). Available from https://www.cdc.gov/tobacco/data_statistics/fact_sheets/economics/econ_facts/index.htm.

Centers for Disease Control, National Center for Chronic Disease Prevention and Health Promotion, Office on Smoking and Health. (2017b). *Health Effects of Cigarette Smoking* (Fast Facts and Fact Sheets). Available from https://www.cdc.gov/tobacco/data_statistics/fact_sheets/health_effects/effects_cig_smoking/index.htm.

Centers for Disease Control, National Center for Chronic Disease Prevention and Health Promotion, Office on Smoking and Health. (2017c). *Secondhand Smoking (SHS) Facts* (Fast Facts and Fact Sheets). Available from https://www.cdc.gov/tobacco/data_statistics/fact_sheets/secondhand_smoke/general_facts/index.htm.

Centers for Disease Control, National Center for Chronic Disease Prevention and Health Promotion, Office on Smoking and Health. (2017d). *Tips from Former Smokers* ® (video). Available from https://www.cdc.gov/tobacco/campaign/tips/resources/videos/index.html.

Centers for Disease Control, National Center for Chronic Disease Prevention and Health Promotion, Office on Smoking and Health. (2017e). *Youth and Tobacco Use* (Fast Facts and Fact Sheets). Available from https://www.cdc.gov/tobacco/data_statistics/fact_sheets/youth_data/tobacco_use/index.htm.

Centers for Disease Control, National Center for Chronic Disease Prevention and Health Promotion, Office on Smoking and Health. (2018). *Burden of Tobacco Use in the U.S.: Current Cigarette Smoking Among U.S. Adults Aged 18 Years and Older.* Available from https://www.cdc.gov/tobacco/campaign/tips/resources/data/cigarette-smoking-in-united-states.html.

Chamberlain, C., O'Mara-Eves, A., Oliver, S., Caird, J. R., Perlen, S. M., Eades, S. J., & Thomas, J. (2013). Psychosocial interventions for supporting women to stop smoking in pregnancy. *The Cochrane Database of Systematic Reviews, 10*, CD001055. https://doi.org/10.1002/14651858.cd001055.pub4.

Chavez, L. J., Ornelas, I. J., Lyles, C. R., & Williams, E. C. (2015). Racial/ethnic workplace discrimination: Association with tobacco and alcohol use. *American Journal of Preventive Medicine, 48*(1), 42–49. https://doi.org/10.1016/j.amepre.2014.08.013.

Contreary, K. A., Chattopadhyay, S. K., Hopkins, D. P., Chaloupka, F. J., Forster, J. L., Grimshaw, V., et al. (2015). Economic impact of tobacco price increases through taxation: A community guide systematic review. *American*

Journal of Preventive Medicine, 49(5), 800–808. https://doi.org/10.1016/j.amepre.2015.04.026.

DeFrain, J., & Asay, S. (Eds.). (2008). *Strong families around the world: Strengths-based research and perspectives*. London and New York: Routledge and Taylor & Francis.

DeFrain, J., & The University of Nebraska-Lincoln Extension Family Research and Writing Team. (2012). *Getting connected, staying connected: Loving one another day by day*. Indianapolis: iUniverse.

Dierker, L. C., Avenevoli, S., Stolar, M., & Merikangas, K. (2014). Smoking and depression: An examination of mechanisms of comorbidity. *American Journal of Psychiatry, 159*(6), 947–953. https://doi.org/10.1176/appi.ajp.159.6.947.

Drake, P., Driscoll, A. K., & Mathews, T. J. (2018). Cigarette smoking during pregnancy: United States, 2016. *NCHS Data Brief, No. 305*. Hyattsville, MD: National Center for Health Statistics.

Durkin, S., Brennan, E., & Wakefield, M. (2012). Mass media campaigns to promote smoking cessation among adults: An integrative review. *Tobacco Control, 21*(2), 127–138. https://doi.org/10.1136/tobaccocontrol-2011-050345.

Eakin, M. N., Rand, C. S., Borrelli, B., Bilderback, A., Hovell, M., & Riekert, K. A. (2014). Effectiveness of motivational interviewing to reduce head start children's secondhand smoke exposure. A randomized clinical trial. *American Journal of Respiratory and Critical Care Medicine, 189*(12), 1530–1537. https://doi.org/10.1164/rccm.201404-0618oc.

Evans-Polce, R. J., Castaldelli-Maia, J. M., Schomerus, G., & Evans-Lacko, S. E. (2015). The downside of tobacco control? Smoking and self-stigma: A systematic review. *Social Science & Medicine, 145*, 26–34. https://doi.org/10.1016/j.socscimed.2015.09.026.

Farrelly, M. C., Loomis, B. R., Han, B., Gfroerer, J., Kuiper, N., Couzens, G. L., et al. (2013). A comprehensive examination of the influence of state tobacco control programs and policies on youth smoking. *American Journal of Public Health, 103*(3), 549–555. https://doi.org/10.2105/ajph.2012.300948.

Gately, I. (2002). *Tobacco: A cultural history of how an exotic plant seduced civilization*. New York: Grove Press.

Gerking, S., & Khaddaria, R. (2012). Perceptions of health risk and smoking decisions of young people. *Health Economics, 21*(7), 865–877. https://doi.org/10.1002/hec.1760.

Gilman, S. L., & Zhou, X. (2004). *Smoke: A global history of smoking*. London: Reaktion.

Haasova, M., Warren, F., Ussher, M., Van Rensburg, K. J., Faulkner, G., Cropley, M., et al. (2014). The acute effects of physical activity on cigarette cravings: Exploration of potential moderators, mediators and physical activity attributes using individual participant data (IPD) meta-analyses. *Psychopharmacology, 231*(7), 1267–1275. https://doi.org/10.1007/s00213-014-3450-4.

Harrald, C., & Watkins, F. (2010). *The cigarette book: The history and culture of smoking*. New York: Skyhorse Publishing.

Huxley, R. R., & Woodward, M. (2011). Cigarette smoking as a risk factor for coronary heart disease in women compared with men: A systematic review and meta-analysis of prospective cohort studies. *The Lancet, 378*(9799), 1297–1305. https://doi.org/10.1016/s0140-6736(11)60781-2.

Iglesias-Rios, L., & Parascandola, M. (2013). A historical review of R.J. Reynolds' strategies for marketing tobacco to Hispanics in the United States. *American Journal of Public Health, 103*(5), e15–e27. https://doi.org/10.2105/ajph.2013.301256.

Jacobs, M., Alonso, A. M., Sherin, K. M., Koh, Y., Dhamija, A., Lowe, A. L., & ACPM Prevention Practice Committee. (2013). Policies to restrict secondhand smoke exposure: American college of preventive medicine position statement. *American Journal of Preventive Medicine, 45*(3), 360–367. https://doi.org/10.1016/j.amepre.2013.05.007.

Jayes, L., Britton, J., Vardavas, C., & Leonardi-Bee, J. (2014). Systematic reviews and meta-analyses on the effects of active and passive smoking on respiratory health outcomes: The SmokeHaz online resource. *The Lancet, 384*(2), S42. https://doi.org/10.1016/s0140-6736(14)62168-1.

Jha, P., Ramasundarahettige, C., Landsman, V., Rostron, B., Thun, M., Anderson, R. N., et al. (2013). 21st-century hazards of smoking and benefits of cessation in the United States. *New England Journal of Medicine, 368*(4), 341–350. https://doi.org/10.1056/nejmsa1211128.

Jones, A. M., Laporte, A., Rice, N., & Zucchelli, E. (2015). Do public smoking bans have an impact on active smoking? Evidence from the UK. *Health Economics, 24*(2), 175–192. https://doi.org/10.1002/hec.3009.

King, B. A., Dube, S. R., & Homa, D. M. (2013). Smoke-free rules and secondhand smoke exposure in homes and vehicles among U.S. adults, 2009–2010. *Preventing Chronic Disease, 10*, e79. https://doi.org/10.5888/pcd10.120218.

Klein, R. (1995). *Cigarettes are sublime*. London: Picador Press. ISBN 0-330-34016-6.

Kluger, R. (1996). *Ashes to ashes: America's hundred-year cigarette war, the public health, and the unabashed triumph of Philip Morris*. New York: Alfred A. Knopf.

Levinson, A. H. (2017). Where the U.S. tobacco epidemic still rages: Most remaining smokers have lower socioeconomic status. *Journal of Health Care for the Poor and Underserved,* 28(1), 11–107. https://doi.org/10.1353/hpu.2017.0012.

Nguyen, S. N., Von Kohorn, I., Schulman-Green, D., & Colson, E. R. (2012). The importance of social networks on smoking: Perspectives of women who quit smoking during pregnancy. *Maternal Child Health Journal, 16*, 1312–1318. https://doi.org/10.1007/s10995-011-0896-4.

Okoli, C. T. C., & Kodet, J. (2015). A systematic review of secondhand tobacco smoke exposure and smoking behaviors: Smoking status, susceptibility, initiation, dependence, and cessation. *Addictive Behaviors, 47*, 22–32.

Olson, D. H., DeFrain, J., & Skogrand, L. (2018). *Marriages and families: Intimacy, diversity, and strengths* (9th ed.). New York: McGraw-Hill Higher Education.

Pacek, L. R., & McClernon, F. J. (2018). Decline in the perceived risk of cigarette smoke between 2006 and 2015: Findings from a U.S. nationally representative sample. *Drug and Alcohol Dependence, 185*, 406–410. doi: https://doi.org/10.1016/j.drugalcdep.2018.01.002.

Slovic, P. (Ed.). (2001). *Smoking: Risk, perception, & policy*. Thousand Oaks, CA: Sage. ISBN 0-7619-2381-0.

Soneji, S., Sargent J., & Tanski, S. (2016). Multiple tobacco product use among US adolescents and young adults. *Tobacco Control, 25*, 174–180. https://doi.org/10.1136/tobaccocontrol-2014-051638.

Stead, L. F., Perera, R., Bullen, C., Mant, D., Hartmann-Boyce, J., Cahill, K., & Lancaster, T. (2012). Nicotine replacement therapy for smoking cessation. *The Cochrane Database of Systematic Reviews, 11*, CD000146. https://doi.org/10.1002/14651858.cd000146.pub4.

Stewart, M. J., Greaves, L., Kushner, K. E., Letourneau, N. L., Spitzer, D. L., & Boscoe, M. (2011). Where there is smoke, there is stress: Low-income women identify support needs and preferences for smoking reduction. *Health Care for Women International, 32*(5), 359–383. https://doi.org/10.1080/07399332.2010.530724.

Szasz, T. (1985). *Ceremonial Chemistry* (Rev, ed.). Holmes Beach, FL: Learning Publications. ISBN 0-918452-83-X.

Tarnoki, A. D., Tarnoki, D. L., Lazar, Z., Karlinger, K., Molnar, A. A., Garami, Z., et al. (2012). Role of genetic factors on smoking habits and secondhand smoke sensitivity: A twin study. *European Respiratory Journal, 40*(Suppl. 56), 4511.

Tsai, Y. W., Chang, L. C., Sung, H. Y., Hu, T. W., & Chiou, S. T. (2015). The impact of smoke-free legislation on reducing exposure to secondhand smoke: Differences across gender and socioeconomic groups. *Tobacco Control, 24*(1), 62–69. https://doi.org/10.1136/tobaccocontrol-2013-051004.

U.S. Department of Health and Human Services. *The Health Consequences of Smoking—50 Years of Progress. A Report of the Surgeon General.* Atlanta: U.S. Department of Health and Human Services, Centers for Disease Control and Prevention, National Center for Chronic Disease Prevention and Health Promotion, Office on Smoking and Health, 2014. Available from https://www.cdc.gov/tobacco/data_statistics/sgr/50th-anniversary/index.htm.

van de Griendt, M. (2008). *Smokin' boys smokin' girls.* English translation by Kumar Jamdagni, Zwolle. B-önnigheim (Germany): Wacher GmbH www.wachter.de. ISBN 978 90 5330 633 8.

Whittaker, R., McRobbie, H., Bullen, C., Borland, R., Rodgers, A., & Gu, Y. (2012). Mobile phone-based interventions for smoking cessation. *Cochrane Database of Systematic Reviews* (11). https://doi.org/10.1002/14651858.cd006611.pub3.

Wilson, L. M., Avila Tang, E., Chander, G., Hutton, H. E., Odelola, O. A., Elf, J. L., et al. (2012). Impact of tobacco control interventions on smoking initiation, cessation, and prevalence: A systematic review. *Journal of Environmental and Public Health, 2012.* https://doi.org/10.1155/2012/961724.

Index

I. Newman and J. DeFrain, *Tobacco Use and Intimate Relationships*,
https://doi.org/10.1007/978-3-319-92579-0

The manufacturer's authorised representative in the EU is Springer Nature Customer Service Centre GmbH, Europaplatz 3, 69115 Heidelberg, Germany. If you have any concerns regarding our products, please contact ProductSafety@springernature.com

Printed and bound by CPI Group (UK) Ltd, Croydon, CR0 4YY
30/09/2026
02225660-0007